The ADHD and AUTISM NUTRITIONAL SUPPLEMENT

Handbook

The Cutting-Edge Biomedical Approach to Treating the Underlying Deficiencies and Symptoms of ADHD and Autism

Dana Godbout Laake, R.D.H., M.S., L.D.N., and Pamela J. Compart, M.D.
Authors of *The Kid-Friendly ADHD and Autism Cookbook*

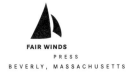

FAIR WINDS
PRESS
BEVERLY, MASSACHUSETTS

In loving memory of our parents:
Ruth and Henry Compart
Dottie and Bill Beers
and
To the children and families we are privileged to serve
Who continue to be our muses and teachers.
We are humbled in your presence.

....

© 2013 Fair Winds Press
Text © 2013 Dana Godbout Laake and Pamela J. Compart

First published in the USA in 2013 by
Fair Winds Press, a member of
Quayside Publishing Group
100 Cummings Center
Suite 406-L
Beverly, MA 01915-6101
www.fairwindspress.com

17 16 15 14 13   1 2 3 4 5

ISBN: 978-1-59233-517-6

Digital edition published in 2013
eISBN: 978-1-61058-616-0

Library of Congress Cataloging-in-Publication Data

Laake, Dana Godbout.
  The ADHD and autism nutritional supplement handbook : the cutting-edge biomedical approach to treating the underlying deficiencies and symptoms of ADHD and autism / Dana Laake and Pamela Compart, M.D.
      pages cm
  Includes bibliographical references and index.
  ISBN 978-1-59233-517-6
  1. Autism in children--Diet therapy--Handbooks, manuals, etc. 2. Asperger›s syndrome in children--Diet therapy--Handbooks, manuals, etc. 3. Attention-deficit hyperactivity disorder--Diet therapy--Handbooks, manuals, etc. I. Compart, Pamela J. II. Title.
  RJ506.A9L317 2013
  618.92'85882--dc23
                          2012037709

Book design by Mighty Media Inc.
Printed and bound in U.S.A.

The information in this book is for educational purposes only. It is not intended to replace the advice of a physician or medical practitioner. Please see your health care provider before beginning any new health program.

Contents

CHAPTER 3: *Getting to Know the Landscape: The Primary Systems, Mechanisms, and Epigenetics*   154

CHAPTER 4: *Tuning the Engine: Nutrients and Their Impact on Impaired Systems and Out-of-Sync Mechanisms*   172

Vitamins 172

CHAPTER 5: *Avoiding Traffic Accidents and Traffic Jams: Toxic Metals and Nutrient/Medication/ Herb/Food Interactions*

CHAPTER 6: *The Right Fuel: An Overview of Special Diets*

Foreword

Nature has provided our bodies and minds with multiple pathways to preserve and enhance the function of our species. We have the capacity for rich social interactions, complex intellectual computations, and rewarding empathetic relationships. Every second in every cell of every human, simultaneous synergistic and intricate interactions facilitate our ability to function as complicated chemical, electrical, and social beings.

As a species, we have a moral imperative to protect and nurture our children. The advent of public health measures and the development of antibiotics have minimized the impact of life-threatening acute infectious illnesses, but they have failed to address the multiple environmental threats that affect the complex synergy of cellular function and increased susceptibility to chronic illness. In many of our children, we have lost the carefully orchestrated symphony that facilitates our body–mind interactions and are left with a noisy cacophony of misdirected cellular messages and disconnected neuronal pathways.

As I write these words, the American Academy of Pediatrics reports that 1 in 6 children now has a developmental, emotional, or behavioral disorder. The latest figures from the Centers for Disease Control and Prevention show that autism spectrum disorders affect 1 in 88 children in the United States (in Utah, where there are widespread screening programs, 1 in 47 children is affected). However, autism spectrum disorders affect the genders unevenly; a staggering 1 in 54 boys is diagnosed with autism in the United States. Furthermore, 54 percent of children have at least one chronic illness.

Our best evidence suggests that combinations of genetic predispositions and environmental exposures conspire to disrupt the innate mechanisms that nature has devised to protect our children. Between 300 and 800 genes are believed to be involved in the expression of autism. Environmental hazards act on the genome in various ways depending upon a specific child's genetic makeup. Although alterations to the genome, whether visible in a chromosomal karyotype or present as a mutation in a single nucleotide, have long been established as causes of disorders, gene expression has been explored more recently for physiological effects. Epigenetics, the study of chemical markers that switch genes on or off, may prove to be a fruitful field for the treatment of complex disorders. The interplay of genetic mutation and epigenetics can generate underlying metabolic, immune, inflammatory, digestive, neurological, and nutritional aberrations, which can be identified through testing and treated appropriately.

The good news is that we have specific, evidence-based strategies that utilize nature's pharmacopoeia to promote the function of disrupted pathways and dysfunctional neurons. The most sophisticated treatment strategies strive to address the unique needs of each individual child from behavioral, educational, medical, metabolic, and nutritional perspectives.

Based upon the abundance of scientific research and drawing on years of experience working with children affected by developmental disorders, Dana Godbout Laake and Pamela Compart have compiled clinically valuable and specific guidelines for therapies that can change the trajectory of children's lives. They describe clinical symptoms and physical signs common in ADHD and autism, providing detailed information about specific nutritional intervention treatment options. They present the systems, mechanisms, and nutritional biochemical science and laboratory testing that serve as the rationale for the recommendations. Also provided are extensive medical and scientific resources and references for those who seek more information.

With the publication of this book, parents and clinicians can find very specific recommendations to guide them on their quest to help a generation of children lead happier and more productive lives. The authors clearly explain why prior recommended allowances and current dietary reference intakes may not meet the nutritional demands of an individual child.

Children with developmental disorders, ADHD, and autism also live with other medical problems. These maladies cause not only physical pain, but also psychological suffering. Parents, teachers, medical practitioners, and others have seen the frustration written on a child's face as he or she yearns to communicate wants and needs, but cannot. For years I have acted upon the belief that it is a moral imperative for adults to seek therapeutic, integrative interventions. This book provides data on nutritional supplementation that can make life with these disorders better.

Elizabeth Mumper, M.D., F.A.A.P.
Advocates for Children
Advocates for Families
Rimland Center for Integrative Medicine, Lynchburg, Virginia
Former Medical Director of the Autism Research Institute

Introduction: Let's Talk About It

The journey of providing supplementation to treat symptoms of Attention Deficit Hyperactivity Disorder (ADHD) and autism may seem like driving through the country on roads devoid of signs and with no available guidebook, map, GPS, or directions. All you know is where you are. You do not know where you are supposed to be going or how to get there. Let us be your tour guides and take this journey together.

If you are reading this book, your life has been touched by ADHD or autism in some way. You may be a parent of a child with ADHD or autism seeking to help your child reach his or her potential, a grandparent who wants to support your child and grandchild, or a concerned friend. You may be a physician who wants to expand your knowledge in a field not yet fully addressed in traditional educational forums. This book is an attempt to address these needs by making nutritional supplements and their use understandable.

We think the most effective approach to treating autism and other behavioral and developmental disorders uses these three tools:

1. Educational placements and therapies (e.g., speech, occupational, behavioral, and social skills therapy)
2. Medication
3. A biomedical approach that is based on laboratory findings and clinical presentation and addresses the person's underlying metabolic, nutritional, and dietary problems

What Is ADHD?

ADHD is the name given to a cluster of symptoms that includes inattention, hyperactivity, and impulsivity. There are three different ADHD subtypes:

- Predominately inattentive
- Predominantly hyperactive-impulsive
- Combined type

For a complete description, see the *Diagnostic and Statistical Manual of Mental Disorders*, 4th ed. (*DSM-IV*).

What Is Autism?

Autism is a developmental disorder affecting communication and social interaction. It is also a clinical diagnosis based on three main areas of symptoms as described in the *DSM-IV*.

1. Qualitative impairments in social interaction
2. Qualitative impairments in communication
3. Restricted, repetitive, and stereotyped patterns of behavior, interests, and activities

TOOLS FOR THE JOURNEY: WHY USE NUTRITIONAL SUPPLEMENTS?

Nutrition is directly related to health and brain function. There is some truth to the saying "you are what you eat." Many children have limited appetites and poor food selection, which lead to them receiving an inadequate amount of nutrients. However, even children with good appetites, a varied diet, and excellent food intake may not be getting enough nutrients to meet their body's specific needs. The goal for all children is to meet each child's specific nutritional needs for optimal brain and body functions.

For children with behavioral and developmental challenges, including autism spectrum disorders and, to a lesser degree, ADHD, body chemistry can be significantly disrupted in ways that require additional nutritional support.

Note that diet and nutrition are not the same. Diet is what you eat. Nutrition is what you eat, digest, absorb, and deliver to the cells, as well as how the cells use the nutrients. There are many steps in this process that can be faulty or inefficient, leading to higher-than-usual nutrient needs. In many cases, diet is woefully insufficient in meeting these exceptional needs, and in these situations, nutritional supplements can be helpful.

As you will learn from this book, the biochemical difficulties, particularly for children on the autism spectrum, can be multilayered and complex. For children with ADHD, the body chemistry disruptions are less severe and less complex. The goal is to provide the nutrients needed by each child, based on specific biochemical needs aimed toward maximizing brain and body function. A child's best prognosis will come from optimal, not marginal, nutritional status. This book is an attempt to make this chemistry more understandable and provide you with practical guidance on how to support your child's body chemistry and, ultimately, brain and body function.

How do you begin to organize your thoughts about this overwhelming amount of material? Sidney Baker, M.D., a renowned functional medicine physician, describes a two-question approach to anyone who is not thriving. Paraphrased here, the two questions are:

1. Are this person's brain and body getting everything that he or she needs to function optimally?
2. Is there something getting into this person's brain and body that is interfering with his or her optimal function?

This is a concise description of functional medicine, an approach to treatment that seeks to improve function regardless of a person's label. The basic approach is to give the body what it needs and get rid of what it doesn't. This is a simple yet elegant premise from which very sophisticated treatment options flow.

Substances that the brain and body need for optimal function include adequate protein, carbohydrates, fats, water, vitamins, minerals, essential fatty acids, and other nutrient cofactors. Problems that can interfere with achieving optimal brain and body function include poor digestion, poor absorption, impaired cellular utilization, food intolerances, yeast or bacterial toxins, histamine from allergies, toxin exposure, certain medications, and toxins generated from the body's own metabolic processes. By providing those elements that the body and brain need and eliminating those that they don't, improvements may appear in language, mood, behavior, attention, cognition, social interaction, digestion, immunity, endurance, coordination, and eye contact. Overall health and well-being are also supported.

Is this Journey Okay for Others? What if I Am Not Sure Whether My Child Has ADHD or Autism—Can this Book Still Be Helpful?

Functional medicine approaches do not require a definitive label or specific diagnosis to be effective. Again, the goal is to improve function and reduce or eliminate problematic symptoms, regardless of a label. Nutritional deficiencies and interfering factors as described previously can be identified and addressed, with the hope of decreasing or eliminating problematic physical, behavioral, neurological, immune, and developmental symptoms.

If you are a parent, you are likely asking yourself the following questions:
- Where do I start?
- Does my child need everything I've read or heard about, and how do I decide what is relevant to him or her?
- Are these supplements safe?
- How do I know how much to give?
- What are the side effects?
- How do I get my child to take the supplements?
- What is safe to do on my own?
- When do I need a specialist (physician, nutritionist, etc.) to guide me?
- Is any testing needed?
- What type of outcome should I expect? How soon should I expect to see changes?

These are all questions you should ask. The goal of treatment is to help your child reach his or her potential in a safe, thoughtful, and coordinated way. This book aims to provide guidance and answers to these questions.

How Do I Start?

Treatment is a multilayered process. Our approach is to start with treatments that have significant benefit with the least likelihood of negative side effects. This book will give you a variety of different ways to start helping your child. The first half of the book is designed to provide practical information on supplements that have been demonstrated to be effective.

Chapter 1.2, "The Quick Start: Six Supplements with the Biggest Benefits and Fewest Side Effects" reviews what we think are the most important supplements for helping overall function. It addresses the most common deficiencies or imbalances and uses supplements with the least likelihood of significant side effects.

"The Quick Start Diet" provides basic guidelines for a healthy organic diet.

Chapter 2, "Moving Forward: Supplementation Based on Specific Signs and Symptoms," provides significant details on eighteen of the most common symptoms noted in ADHD and autism. Included are the most important supplements for treating those symptoms along with supplement type, specific instructions regarding dosing, side effects, and more.

The second half of the book provides explanations of the underlying primary systems, mechanisms, and epigenetics followed by detailed chapters on specific vitamins, minerals, and other nutrients. Additional sections address toxic metals, nutrient/drug/diet interactions, and special diets.

This book is not intended to be a substitute for working with a professional who has expertise in biomedical treatments (such as a physician, dietitian/nutritionist, naturopath, nurse practitioner, physician assistant, or nurse). It is ideal to have a practitioner evaluate your child and determine, through clinical judgment and a variety of basic and specialized tests, what your child's biochemical strengths and weaknesses are and which specific nutrients and doses are most appropriate. Individualizing your child's treatment program will result in the best chance for the most successful outcome.

CHAPTER 1

The Journey Begins: Getting Started and Supplementing Safely

There are many ways to determine which supplements to use for your child. Lab tests, an important tool in diagnosis and treatment, are discussed under the individual nutrient chapters beginning in chapter 4. Another critical way is to look at those symptoms and conditions (behaviors, delays, physical signs, health issues, medications, toxic exposures) that interfere with your child's optimal brain and body functioning and then determine which supplements may be helpful. We have designed this section to take you through the thought process we use when we see children in our offices.

Recommendations are not a substitute for medical advice. Rather, it is ideal to work with a health care practitioner trained in functional medicine to evaluate and individualize the treatment plan for your child, including specific supplements, optimal dosing, and the order of implementation. However, we recognize that depending on where you live, you may not have access to these types of health care practitioners. Even if you do, the health care practitioner may have a long waiting list or not be affordable. We have written this book with the hope of helping you start using supplements in a safe and thoughtful way for your child.

■ 1.1 Nutrition 101: Terminology, Principles, Recommendations, and Supplementation

Safety First: Do No Harm

Without a specific health care practitioner's guidance and/or lab testing, it is even more important to be vigilant about dosing supplements in a safe way. If a little is good, more is not necessarily better and in fact may be harmful. The recommendations in this section are not the Dietary Reference Intakes/Recommended Dietary Allowances (DRIs/RDAs) that are designed to apply only to healthy individuals who are not taking medications or who do not have one or more of the following: genetic conditions, restricted intakes, poor digestion, poor absorption, metabolic inefficiencies, nutritional deficiencies, excess toxic burden, and other health conditions.

Instead, the dosing guidelines we offer are the maximum we recommend if you are doing this on your own. Testing becomes critical when high doses are used. For some supplements, we have recommended that you do not use them without a health care practitioner's guidance.

No Speeding: How to Supplement—Start Low and Go Slow

For all supplements, we recommend that you start one new supplement at a time three to seven days apart to identify any side effects. Start at a low dose and increase the dose slowly. In general, we recommend starting at one-quarter of the goal dose and increasing by one-quarter of the dose every few days until you reach the goal dose or the maximum tolerated dose.

Depending on how many biochemical inefficiencies or nutritional deficiencies your child has, you may or may not see a benefit from each individual supplement. Some children may not see a benefit until a sufficient number of inefficiencies or deficits are addressed. Again, having a health care practitioner working with you who can do lab testing to uncover your child's specific biochemical issues is ideal and results in the greatest potential benefit.

All listed signs and symptoms may not be present in your child. This also applies to side effects. Your child may have an unusual or unreported side effect. If you think a supplement is making your child worse, decrease it to see whether the symptoms improve, or stop it if the negative symptoms continue.

A caveat on dosing: In this book dosing for each supplement is the total daily dose, unless otherwise stated. So if you see different symptoms that also require the same supplement, do not go over the total daily dose. For example, if your child has hyperactivity, one recommendation may be magnesium at a dose of 200 mg/day. If your child also has constipation, that section may recommend magnesium at 200 mg/day. Your child's magnesium dose should be a total of 200 mg, *not* 400 mg.

Natural, Synthetic, and Artificial Nutrient Forms

Many factors can affect each nutritional supplement's ability to function optimally. The right nutrient form must be taken in and then digested and absorbed by the digestive tract, transported to the tissues, taken up by the cells, and finally be used by the cells to provide function. Function is the bottom line. Also important are the effects of nutrient interactions with other nutrients, foods, herbs, medications, and toxins.

Nutrients occur in a variety of forms that vary in their absorption and utilization. Nutritional supplements may be natural, synthetic, or artificial.

Natural forms are naturally occurring nutrients that:
- Are food-based and can be extracted from food sources
- Contain natural nutrient cofactors along with the given nutrient
- Are lower in microgram, milligram, gram, and unit measures
- Are less concentrated and usually require taking more substance to deliver a specific nutrient amount
- Can cause reactions depending upon food sources

Synthetic forms are synthesized in the lab and
- Contain active sites identical to the natural forms
- Are usually less expensive than naturally occurring forms
- Are more concentrated and usually require taking less substance than naturally occurring forms
- Are often used when therapeutic/high doses are required

Artificial varieties refer to non-natural nutrient forms that are
- Not the forms best used by the body
- May be much less effective than other forms and, in some cases, harmful

Elemental Nutrients versus Nutrient Compounds

Unlike vitamins and amino acids, minerals occur in many types of compound forms such as calcium carbonate, magnesium citrate, zinc picolinate, and more. The elemental amount is the amount of a nutrient in the compound that is available for absorption by the body. For example, zinc citrate is 35 percent zinc, so that 100 mg of zinc citrate provides 35 mg of elemental zinc.

Forms that result in the highest elemental amount may not be forms that are well absorbed or have a high availability for use. There is a range of effectiveness in supplement functions based upon their forms.

In chapter 4, we discuss specific supplements in detail, including the best forms to utilize. Read the supplement labels to determine the type of supplement.

Nutrient Absorption Rates Vary to Maintain Homeostasis and Prevent Toxicity

Body nutrient levels are regulated by absorption, metabolism, and elimination rates. Nutrient absorption rates increase when there are higher needs based upon one or both of the following:
- Low tissue levels, which means there is not enough of the nutrient in the body to meet all of the body's functional needs. We refer to this as the "bank account" of nutrients—what is stored in the tissues.
- Functional deficiency. Even if the nutrient "bank account" is excellent, function may still be poor because of antagonists present and/or defects in cell enzymes and metabolism.

Nutrient absorption rates will decrease when the need declines because of optimal tissue levels and/or good functional efficiency. In addition, the level of intake influences absorption rates. Specifically:
- Absorption rates are higher when small levels of the nutrient are taken in.
- Absorption rates decline when high doses are taken in at one time.

This is the basis for dividing a full daily dose into two or three divided doses to provide the opportunity for the body to absorb what it needs. Elimination of nutrients (and toxins) via breath, urine, feces, and sweat is an additional "safety valve" for preventing excess levels in the body.

All of these mechanisms are the body's way of achieving balance, which is referred to as homeostasis. It is why the safety range of supplements is so broad, and why toxicity is rare. However, there are still individuals who can develop toxicities based upon differences in how nutrients are absorbed, metabolized, stored, and eliminated.

In addition, there are many kinds of interactions among nutrients, foods, medications, and herbs. These interactions can increase or decrease medication effectiveness and also impede nutrient absorption and availability. We provide more detailed information in chapter 5.

DRI/RDA Recommendations versus Individualized Recommendations

The Dietary Reference Intake, or DRI, is a system of nutrient recommendations developed by the Food and Nutrition Board (FNB) at the independent, nonprofit Institute of Medicine. The DRI is a set of reference values used to plan and assess nutrient intakes of most healthy people. These values vary by age, gender, and life stage, and include the following:

- Recommended Dietary Allowance (RDA), which is "the average daily dietary nutrient intake level sufficient to meet the nutrient requirements of nearly all (97 to 98 percent) healthy individuals in a particular life stage and gender group." It is calculated from an Estimated Average Requirement.
- Adequate Intake, which is determined when there is insufficient evidence to establish an RDA. It is based on levels assumed to be adequate based on estimates of nutrient intake by apparently healthy people.
- Tolerable Upper Intake Level, which is "the highest average daily nutrient intake level that is likely to pose *no* risk of adverse health effects to almost all individuals in the general population."

Source: Food and Nutrition Board, Institute of Medicine of the National Academies. Dietary Reference Intakes (2005) the National Academies Press, p. 48, www.nap.edu.

The FNB acknowledges that the recommendations are not intended for individuals with specific health conditions requiring medical care. Defining healthy can begin by identifying disease prevalence statistics. More than 74 percent of the U.S. population has one or more major chronic disease conditions; the DRIs apply to a small percentage of the population—less than 26 percent. The DRIs do not apply to individuals with identified specific nutritional needs based upon genetics, medical history, clinical presentation, laboratory findings, digestion, absorption, chemical and toxic exposures, lifestyle, diet, stressors, medications, and acute conditions. The concept we discuss is treatment based upon each person's biochemical individuality.

"Therapeutic" is the term used to describe the dosing needed to meet the individual's optimal nutrient requirement and to treat deficiencies and metabolic defects resulting from the environmental/lifestyle impact on that individual's unique gene variants. This level may vary according to the individual's compliance and progress.

The goal in supplementation is to identify each individual's specific nutritional needs and provide the nutrient intakes appropriate to achieving optimal nutrition in that individual.

Supplement Regulation and Safety

Dietary supplements are regulated by the Food and Drug Administration (FDA) and Federal Trade Commission as well as state governments. Extensive regulations govern the manufacturing, labeling, and marketing of dietary supplements. Under the Dietary Supplement Health and Education Act (DSHEA), manufacturers are responsible for ensuring that products are safe. DSHEA permits the FDA to have enforcement authority, including the ability to remove from the market products the agency deems unsafe, an "imminent hazard," or a "significant or unreasonable risk" of causing illness or injury.

The FDA established comprehensive regulations called Good Manufacturing Practices (GMP) that apply to pharmaceuticals and supplements. Regulations cover buildings and facilities, equipment, personnel, raw materials, production, laboratory controls, records, labeling, complaints, and recalls. There are provisions under DSHEA that protect consumers from potentially unsafe products.

Manufacturers and distributors of dietary supplements must record, investigate, and forward reports to the FDA if they receive notice of any serious adverse events associated with the use of their products. The FDA evaluates these reports and any other adverse events reported directly by health care providers or consumers to identify potential risks. Note the comparison of adverse/serious events from supplements and prescriptions taken in 2010:

- Of more than 50 percent of the population taking one or more supplements, a reported 60 billion doses, there were 1,275 adverse events reported.
- Of the 48 percent of the population taking one or more prescription drugs (3.8 billion prescriptions), there were 759,000 adverse events reported.

Comparison of deaths from supplements with deaths from pharmaceuticals:
- Supplements: 2 to 5 per year (the risk for death from supplements is 0.0001 percent)
- Pharmaceuticals: up to 160,000 per year

Beyond GMP measures that ensure supplement safety, supplement companies can formulate their products using the latest clinical research and include optimal nutrient forms and therapeutic dosage levels. Manufacturers can also produce supplements that are hypoallergenic by excluding binders, fillers, dyes, coatings, and common allergens such as soy, gluten, dairy, and corn. Health care professionals can provide specific product recommendations and doses that are best suited to the individual's needs.

Tips on Getting Your Child to Take Supplements

No matter how good a supplement is, it is of no benefit if your child refuses to take it. Children are generally not willing to take supplements simply because they are good for them; they need them to either taste good or be hidden in a food or liquid so that they are undetectable. The following are suggestions for giving supplements:

- If your child cannot swallow pills, you may need to open capsules and crush tablets, mixing the powder into foods or liquids. You can add powders or liquids to juices, smoothies, syrup, pudding, ketchup, yogurt, and sorbets.
- Chocolate syrup or peanut butter (or other nut butters) are good choices for hiding fish oils. The fat in these products coats the taste buds, which better masks any negative taste. The consistency of these foods is also good for blending oils.
- Some powders will not dissolve fully in liquids, and children will reject a drink with particles. Some will reject powder in liquid simply based on seeing it; using sippy cups or opaque cups may help with this.
- Chewable tablets can be crushed and mixed in food or liquid.
- Most supplements cannot be added to foods and heated. However, they can be added to warm foods after they are cooked.
- Powdered supplements can be added to ketchup (use gluten-free ketchup when needed).
- Powders or liquids can be added to homemade ice pops made from juice and frozen. This may work well for some stronger tasting vitamins, such as B vitamins.
- Flavoring liquids are available commercially or from compounding pharmacists.
- Some nutrients are absorbable through the skin (e.g., zinc, glutathione, vitamin D). If not commercially available, a compounding pharmacist can make specific transdermal preparations.

If your child is able to swallow pills, the following tips may make it easier:

- Capsules are lighter than water because of the air trapped inside. To best swallow capsules, place the capsule in the mouth, take a sip of liquid, and tip the head forward. This allows the capsule to float upward and more easily reach the back of the throat.
- Tablets are heavier than water. To best swallow tablets, place the tablet in the mouth, take a sip of water, and tip the head back.

■ *1.2 The Quick Start: Six Supplements with the Biggest Benefits and Fewest Side Effects*

Where do you start: with supplements or diet? There is no absolute right answer to this. If your child is already on a healthy diet and/or special diet and not on supplements, then continue while you begin adding supplements. If your child is already on supplements but not on any type of healthy or special diet, expand the supplements as you change the diet.

If you have not attempted any diets or supplements, begin with the supplements as you also improve the diet quality based on the advice in the second section of this chapter. Our experience is that when children begin supplementing, there can be improvements in behavior, cooperation, sensory issues, and cognition—all of which can make it easier to facilitate change and expand the diet, including moving to a core organic healthy diet and, if needed, one of the special diets.

THE QUICK START SUPPLEMENTS

There are many ways to approach introducing supplements to your child. One option is to start with a core group of supplements that provide the greatest overall benefit with the fewest side effects. This chapter contains, in order of appearance, the six supplements that we have observed usually provide the broadest benefits:

A. Magnesium

B. Vitamin D

C. Zinc

D. Essential omega-3 fatty acids

E. Probiotics

F. Multiple vitamin–mineral (multivitamin)

We describe each of these supplements, including the basis and benefits for the supplement selection, dosing guidelines, and possible side effects. More detailed explanations of each of these supplements appear in chapter 4.

▶ A. MAGNESIUM

Magnesium is needed for more than 350 biomedical reactions in the body, affecting 75 percent of enzyme functions. Magnesium is critical to neurotransmitter function, core energy metabolism, hormone metabolism, protein synthesis, cell membrane function, blood pressure regulation, calcium metabolism, muscle function, bowel function, and memory.

A person deficient in magnesium may experience neuromuscular excitability, which can lead to hyperactivity, distractibility, impulsivity, muscle spasms, and poor sleep quality. Magnesium is a common nutritional deficiency in children with ADHD or autism and in the general population.

Magnesium has calming effects on the nervous system. When magnesium is deficient, the following symptoms can occur:

- ADHD symptoms, including hyperactivity, inattention, and impulsivity
- Mood dysregulation, including depression
- Cognitive problems
- Anxiety, fears
- Emotional overreactions
- Irritability
- Aggression
- Poor self-regulation
- Muscle spasms
- Sleep disruption
- Restless sleep (tossing and turning)
- Nightmares, night terrors
- Memory loss
- Excessive sighing or yawning
- Sound or light sensitivity
- Constipation
- Neuromuscular excitability, easy startle, or brisk reflexes
- Seizures

What to Do and How to Do It—Magnesium Supplements

The type of magnesium used often depends on whether you are also trying to treat bowel problems. Magnesium tends to have a laxative effect, depending upon the form it comes in.
- Gentle (less laxative) stool effect: chelates, aspartates, glycinates, and gluconates
- Laxative stool effect: citrates, chlorides, and sulfates

MAGNESIUM TOTAL DAILY GOAL DOSING

AGE	DOSE	FREQUENCY	TOTAL DAILY DOSE FROM ALL SOURCES
2 to 5	100 mg	1 or 2 times per day	200 mg
6 to 10	100 mg	2 to 3 times per day	300 mg
11 +	100 to 150 mg	2 to 3 times per day	450 mg

- Start at one-quarter to one-half of the recommended dose and increase the dose gradually every one to two days.
- Magnesium can cause loose stools or diarrhea.

- Watch for possible side effects and decrease the dose accordingly.
- If symptoms improve at lower than the goal dose, you may not need to increase the dose further.
- For higher-than-recommended doses, consult with a skilled health care practitioner.

How to Get Magnesium from Your Diet

Vegetables, especially greens, are rich in magnesium. Other good sources include beans, nuts, seeds, and fruits. Children with picky appetites typically have low intakes of magnesium. Because of taste and food aversions, common among those with ADHD and autism, it is difficult to coax children into consuming these foods.

We recommend hiding vegetable and fruit purees in meatballs, spaghetti sauce, and fruit smoothies. This "Trojan Horse Technique" is described in our book, *The Kid-Friendly ADHD & Autism Cookbook*.

What Side Effects Should I Watch for?

The main side effect of magnesium is loose stools. When this occurs, cut back on the dose. Because loose stools deplete magnesium, toxicity from oral doses is extremely rare. Magnesium is self-limiting. It is extremely unusual to have behavioral side effects from magnesium, though we occasionally see children who are extremely sensitive to magnesium (even the magnesium used as filler in capsules). This is another reason to increase the dose gradually.

Calcium intake should be adequate when taking magnesium. Excess magnesium intake can lower calcium, and excess calcium intake can lower magnesium. It is important to have balance. If your child is not getting sufficient calcium from diet, a calcium supplement is indicated.

CALCIUM TOTAL DAILY GOAL DOSING

AGE	DOSE	FREQUENCY	TOTAL DAILY DOSE FROM ALL SOURCES
2 to 5	250 mg	2 times per day	500 mg
6 to 10	250 mg	3 times per day	750 mg
11 +	500 to 600 mg	2 times per day	1,000 to 1,200 mg

▶ B. VITAMIN D

Vitamin D is necessary for calcium absorption and bone health. It is also important for cognitive function, immunity, skin health, mood, and fetal, infant, and child development. It is also a common deficiency. Risk factors for the development of vitamin D deficiency include inadequate sun exposure, use of sunblock, darker skin pigmentation, obesity, breast feeding, low dietary intake, and fat malabsorption.

Vitamin D deficiency contributes to the following symptoms and clinical conditions:

- Developmental delays and learning disabilities
- Delayed tooth eruption
- Profuse sweating
- Eczema or other skin conditions
- Chronic chapped lips
- Frequent infections
- Rickets—signs can include bowed legs or knock-knees, deformed skull

  Vitamin D Supplements
- Vitamin D$_3$ is available in capsules, tablets, and liquids.
- The micellized version of vitamin D$_3$ is a water-soluble form of vitamin D that is well absorbed and especially useful in malabsorption conditions.
- Vitamin D$_3$ (cholecalciferol) is the best form to utilize for supplementation.
- Vitamin D$_2$ (ergocalciferol) converts to vitamin D$_3$ and is less effective long term.
- The oil and micellized forms are preferred over the dry forms.

A GUIDE TO VITAMIN D$_3$ SUPPLEMENTS

VITAMIN D$_3$ (CHOLECALCIFEROL)	AMOUNT	COMMENTS
Vitamin D drops made by *Carlson, Nordic Naturals*	400 IU/drop	Easy to give
Vitamin D$_3$ capsules	400 IU/capsule	There are capsules from 1,000 to 5,000 IU. Use these only under the care of a health care practitioner.
Micellized vitamin D$_3$ made by *Klaire, Biotics Bio-D-Mulsion*	400 IU/drop	Biotics Bio-D-Mulsion is 2,000-IU drops. Use this only under the care of a health care practitioner.
Vitamin D$_3$ in with omega-3		See essential omega-3 fatty acids on page 24.

VITAMIN D TOTAL DAILY GOAL DOSING

AGE	DOSE	FREQUENCY
2 to 5	400 to 600 IU	Daily
6 to 10	600 to 800 IU	Daily
11 +	800 to 2,000 IU	Daily

- The total daily dose includes all sources such as D from cod liver oil and multiple vitamins, listed in section 4.2 Vitamin D$_3$.
- Have blood testing for vitamin D (25-hydroxy vitamin D) to guide dosing. The optimal goal blood level is 60 to 80 ng/ml.
- Adequate vitamin A intake must be maintained. See the vitamin A recommendations on page 22.
- Higher doses may be required due to poor absorption or lab findings. This should be accomplished with a skilled health care practitioner.

Quick Start: Vitamin D

What Side Effects Should I Watch for?

At the doses recommended, there are typically no side effects. However, if high doses are used long term, there can be nausea and joint pain.

What Else Should I Know?

Food sources include liver, fish and fish oils, and egg yolks. Vitamin D is manufactured in unprotected skin by sun exposure (UVB light). In twenty minutes, the body can manufacture 10,000 IU. Vitamin D_3 is a common deficiency, more prevalent in those who are not exposed to summer sun and those with darker skin color. Supplementation has become an important source of vitamin D_3.

When taking vitamin D, ensure adequate vitamin A intake. Make sure that the total vitamin A intake from cod liver oil, a multiple vitamin–mineral supplement, and additional vitamin A, does not exceed the following doses:

AGE	VITAMIN A DAILY DOSE
2 to 3	1,250 IU
4 to 5	1,250 to 2,500 IU
6 to 10	2,500 to 3,500 IU
11 +	3,500 to 5,000 IU

▶ C. ZINC

There are more than 300 zinc-dependent enzymes in the body. Zinc is important for brain development, gene expression, amino acid metabolism, toxic metal metabolism, epithelial integrity, growth, development, muscle tone, glucose control, digestion, methylation, vision, auditory processing, language processing, and sensory processing. Zinc is also part of the insulin molecule and necessary for vitamin A transport and availability. Zinc deficiency is very common in children with autism and is not uncommon in children with ADHD.

Zinc deficiency can contribute to the following symptoms:

- Picky eating
- Poor eye contact (because of poor vitamin A absorption)
- Pica (eating nonfood substances)
- Sensory processing disorder
- Delays in growth or language
- Skin conditions (eczema, dermatitis, rashes)
- Low muscle tone
- Inflammation and infections
- White lines on nails
- Elevated toxic metals

Zinc Deficiency and Picky Appetite

Deficiency can cause a loss of taste at the taste bud level and also affects perception of taste in the brain. Once taste is diminished or lost, many foods can become unpalatable and even offensive. As zinc status declines, taste perception decreases and aversions increase, especially to vegetables and often to specific textures, colors, and smells. Some children will even gag at the sight of a food that is offensive to them.

Perception is reality, and the child is responding reasonably to the taste perceived. The child then limits choices to a few foods such as sweets, pasta, breads, cold cereals, macaroni and cheese, and ice cream. Some even prefer stronger tasting or spicier foods in an attempt to detect enough taste to make the food tolerable. Other children will simply avoid the unpalatable foods.

What Else You Should Know about Zinc

Zinc is necessary for the function of retinol-binding protein, which transports vitamin A from the liver to the tissues where the vitamin A is utilized. For this reason, zinc deficiency is the main cause of vitamin A deficiency.

Zinc affects external epithelial tissues such as the skin and the epithelial internal mucosal tissues of the mouth, nasal cavities, sinuses, digestive tract, and more. Zinc impacts skin health in two ways: directly from its function in skin integrity, and indirectly through its role in transporting vitamin A.

Zinc's effect on vision is also direct and indirect. The retina contains high levels of zinc, which has a pivotal role in dark adaptation and macular health. Indirectly, zinc affects vision via its transport of vitamin A into the retina where it is utilized.

Zinc Supplements

Zinc is available in liquid and capsule form and as a transdermal lotion. The choice of which to use can depend on a number of factors such as tolerance for oral zinc, which can cause nausea, or use of acid-suppressing medications, which impair zinc absorption.

- Well tolerated: gluconates, chelates, citrates, acetates, picolinates, chlorides, and bisglycinates.
- Strong taste, needs disguising: sulfates.
- Least effective: zinc oxide and zinc carbonate.
- Topical zinc lotions, for those unable to tolerate oral zinc. Avoid the zinc nasal spray as it can decrease the sense of smell.

ZINC TOTAL DAILY GOAL DOSING

AGE	DOSE	FREQUENCY	TOTAL DAILY DOSE FROM ALL SOURCES
2 to 5	5 to 10 mg	1 or 2 times per day	10 to 20 mg
6 to 10	10 mg	2 times per day	20 mg
11 +	10 to 15 mg	2 times per day	20 to 30 mg

For optimal oral absorption, an empty stomach is best, but it may not be feasible if nausea occurs. Large doses can cause gastric discomfort, nausea, and inhibit the digestive enzyme DPP-IV (digests opioids from gluten, casein). In addition:

- Avoid or limit giving oral zinc at the same time as interfering nutrients such as calcium, iron, folate, and phosphorylated nutrients (R5P, P5P, phosphatidylcholine); this may not always be feasible.
- If using topical zinc lotion, consider a lotion by Kirkman Labs (22 mg of zinc per scoop, which is ⅛ teaspoon). Apply lotion to parts of the body that have more muscle than fat. Muscle has a rich blood supply that enhances absorption. Apply the lotion to shoulders, back, or calves and massage in thoroughly. If using other topical supplements, do not mix the lotions.
- Zinc excess can lower copper levels. Copper levels need to be maintained.
- If unable to do blood testing, use the Zinc Tally Taste Test for evaluating progress with zinc supplementation. See page 213.
- Higher doses may be required because of malabsorption, antacid use, toxic metals, or lab findings. This should be accomplished with the help of a skilled health care practitioner.
- Without blood testing, these dosing ranges should not be exceeded without the advice of a health care practitioner. The type of testing is critical. Red blood cell zinc is more sensitive and reliable than plasma or serum measures.

▶ D. ESSENTIAL OMEGA-3 FATTY ACIDS

Essential fatty acids are not manufactured in the body and must be consumed. Omega-3 and omega-6 are the two types of essential fatty acids. Omega-3 includes the precursor source alpha-linolenic acid, or ALA, and direct sources eicosapentaenoic acid (EPA) and docosahexaenoic acid (DHA). Omega-6 includes the precursor linoleic acid and direct source gamma-linolenic acid.

Omega-3 fatty acids help keep cell walls flexible rather than rigid, which in turn helps cells function optimally. EPA is most helpful for skin and hair health and immune function. Approximately 60 percent of the dry weight of the brain is composed of fat, including cholesterol and fatty acids. Omega-3 DHA is a critical structural component of the human brain, retina, and nerves affecting cognition, vision, mood, and behavior. In the brain, omega-3 fatty acid deficiency can result in less than optimal transmission of messages. Both are important and are best taken in combination. A lack of sufficient omega-3 fatty acids, particularly EPA, contributes to:

- Skin conditions, such as eczema, dermatitis, rashes, cradle cap, and keratosis pilaris ("chicken skin")
- Mucosal tissue problems such as: gingivitis in the mouth, rhinitis in the nasal cavities, sinusitis in the sinuses, and digestive tract gastritis, colitis, and more
- Poor hair quality
- Immune dysfunction
- Hard earwax

- Excessive thirst
- Cracking or peeling nails

A lack of sufficient omega-3 fatty acids, particularly DHA, contributes to:
- Developmental delays, including poor motor development
- Language and communication delays
- Impaired cognitive function
- Mood and behavioral disorders
- ADHD symptoms
- Vision dysfunction

The ratio range of omega-6:omega-3 intake should be from 1:1 to 4:1. The standard American diet is omega-6 excessive at 16:1. Excessive omega-6 intake and insufficient omega-3 increases inflammation, cardiovascular disease, cancer, and autoimmunity.

The best food source of omega-3 fatty acids is seafood. Large "steak" fish such as tuna, bluefish, and swordfish are highest in mercury, PCBs, and other toxins and should be avoided, whereas sardines are among the safest. See the website of the Environmental Working Group, www.ewg.org, for more information.

For omega-3 supplements for communication, language, attention, focus, behavior, mood, eye contact, and hyperactivity:
- Choose supplements with DHA amount equal to or greater than the EPA.
- Use only direct source EPA and DHA, which is more efficient than flaxseed source ALA.
- Use toxin-free supplements: pharmaceutical grade or molecular distillation to remove toxins.

EPA is more effective for omega-3 supplements for skin, hair, nails, mucosal tissues, immunity, and inflammation. Flaxseed oil is not an efficient source of EPA.

The types of omega-3 supplements available in capsules, liquids, emulsions, and chewables (see section 4.15 Essential Omega-3 Fatty Acids for specific products) include the following:
- Cod liver oils or emulsions (contain varying amounts of vitamins A and D)
- Fish oils with EPA and DHA (most have more EPA than DHA)
- Fish oils higher in DHA
- Vegetarian ALA flaxseed oil (not efficiently converted to EPA, DHA) is not recommended as a good source of EPA and DHA
- Vegetarian algae-source DHA only is ideal for those allergic to seafood

OMEGA-3 EPA AND DHA TOTAL DAILY GOAL DOSING

AGE	EPA	DHA	FREQUENCY
2 to 5	200 to 400 mg	200 to 400 mg	Daily with food
6 to 10	500 to 650 mg	400 to 500 mg	Daily with food
11 +	500 to 800 mg	500 to 650 mg	Daily with food

Quick Start: Omega-3 Fatty Acids

- Include the amount of vitamin A and vitamin D found in omega-3 oils as part of the total daily dose of those vitamins. Also see the vitamin A recommendations listed on page 21.
- Higher doses of omega-3 fatty acids should only be given under the guidance of a skilled health care practitioner.

What Side Effects Should I Watch for?
Side effects to fish oils are unusual. Some fish oils contain ingredients to which children with food allergies or sensitivities may react. For example, Coromega products contain egg, and some fish oils contain soy. Some children may develop loose stools from fish oils. At high doses, fish oils can affect platelet function and may result in easy bruising. However, this is uncommon.

Because omega-3 fatty acids may affect platelet function (relevant to blood clotting), it is advisable to stop fish oils before elective surgeries or procedures, similar to stopping medications that may affect platelet function. The usual recommendation is to stop for three to five days before the procedure and for two to five days after, depending on the type of surgery. Check with your physician or dentist to determine a more specific recommendation for your child.

▶ E. PROBIOTICS

Probiotics are beneficial live microorganisms called the microbiome, found throughout the body, including in the intestinal tract. There are more than 100 trillion "good bacteria" in the body with 500 to 1,000 different species (forty to fifty of which are main species) in the human gut. They maintain healthy flora, prevent overgrowth of harmful pathogens and yeast, and produce healthy nutrients. For a complete listing of probiotic benefits, see sections 4.16 Probiotics and 2.18 Yeast Overgrowth.

Probiotic supplements:
- May be in single strain to multistrain cultures (*Lactobacillus, Bifidobacterium, Streptococcus, Saccharomyces*)
- Should contain live strains, be stored in freezers prior to use, be shipped on ice, and be stored in refrigerator once opened
- Should be hypoallergenic (containing no milk, casein, gluten, soy, corn, or additives)

Types of supplements:
- *Bifidus infantis* or bifido complexes (for infants)
- *Lactobacillus acidophilus*
- *Lactobacillus/Bifidus* combinations
- Expanded combinations with multiple strains
- *Saccharomyces boulardii* (a beneficial yeast)

Examples of supplement brands:
- UltraBifidus Dairy Free (15 billion/ 1/2 teas) by Metagenics
- *Lactobacillus acidophilus* (3 billion/cap) by Kirkman Labs and Klaire Labs
- Pro-Bio Gold with or without Inulin (20 billion/cap) by Kirkman Labs
- Pro-Bio Chewable Wafer (20 billion/wafer) by Kirkman Labs

PROBIOTIC TOTAL DAILY GOAL DOSING

AGE	DOSE IN CFUS	FREQUENCY
1 to 2	1 to 5 billion	Begin with single bifidobacteria product Expand to mixed cultures for infants, especially if formula fed
3 to 5	5 to 10 billion	In two divided doses
6 to 10	10 to 20 billion	In two divided doses
11 +	10 to 50 billion	In two divided doses

- Start low and increase slowly to try to avoid die-off side effects (see page 59).
  - For products with 5 to 10 billion bacteria, start with one-quarter to one-half capsule once daily and increase by one-quarter to one-half capsule every two to three days until goal dose is reached or die-off symptoms develop.
  - For higher dose probiotics, start with one-quarter capsule and increase by one-quarter capsule every two to three days.
- Probiotics are best taken with mild-temperature food and can also be taken on an empty stomach
- If taking antibiotics, wait at least one hour to give probiotics.
- Consult with a health care practitioner for guidance in using higher dose probiotics.

▶ F. MULTIPLE VITAMIN–MINERAL (MULTIVITAMIN)

In ADHD and autism, there are two seemingly contradictory goals in the nutritional approach:
1. To calm down self-stimulatory behaviors (e.g., hand flapping, finger flicking, etc.), hyperactivity, insomnia, perseverations, aggression, anxiety, and impulsivity
2. To stimulate cognition, language, and communication

Our clinical experience shows that when supplements are used to increase cognition, language, learning, and focus, there may also be an increase in hyperactivity and perseverations. By achieving the calming aspects first, the eventual cognitive stimulation will be less challenging.

The appropriate multiple vitamin–mineral combination can provide a good balance of nutrients that can be synergistic, improving each other's digestion, absorption, and utilization. Although many professionals may recommend starting with a multivitamin as the first supplement, we have chosen to include it after the basic five have been tried because:

- Starting with singular nutrients allows the ability to observe both tolerance and improvements.
- The supplements selected are most likely to achieve improvement without negative effects.
- The singular nutrients selected are most likely to:
  — Reduce self-stimulatory behaviors, perseverations, and hyperactivity
  — Improve sleep patterns
  — Improve attention and focus
  — Improve digestion and nutrient absorption
  — Set the stage for better tolerance of supplements that will improve cognition and language
- In a multiple vitamin, there are set levels of nutrients, some of which may be too low and others too high.
- B vitamins, present in most multiple vitamins, can cause hyperactivity, irritability, and/or sleep disruption in some children and may not be tolerated well initially, but the vitamins may become useful after the core nutrients are taken.

Multiple Vitamin–Mineral Supplements

There are many good multiple vitamin–mineral combinations available as baseline supplements or as more therapeutic selections for ADHD and autism. The supplements we recommend are free of milk casein; gluten; artificial additives, flavors, and colors; environmental impurities and toxins; pesticides; and sweeteners. They may include incremental amounts of soy (a vitamin E source) and corn. They include the most effective form and combination of the nutrients and provide a good baseline supplementation of vitamins and minerals.

There are three groups of multiples. Use the most appropriate, based upon your child's level of sensitivities and history of reactions to multiple vitamin-minerals. The three groups are:

1. Basic multiples with complete vitamins and minerals for those who need the A and D in the multiple and tolerate B vitamins.
2. Basic multiples without A and D. Vitamins A and D may not be needed if already being supplemented (separately or in cod liver oil). These are for children who tolerate B vitamins.
3. Basic multiples without A, D, and B vitamins. Vitamin A and D may not be needed if already being supplemented (separately or in cod liver oil). These are for children who are sensitive to B vitamins or become irritable or hyperactive as a result.

Capsuled supplements may be emptied into food, fruit sauce, or smoothies if your child cannot swallow capsules.

HOW TO DOSE MULTIPLE VITAMIN–MINERAL SUPPLEMENTS

BASIC MULTIPLES WITH COMPLETE VITAMINS AND MINERALS	AGE	DOSING WITH MEALS
Syndion capsules made by *Yasoo* *Includes folinic acid, choline, inositol, CoQ$_{10}$,* *N-A-cysteine*	2 to 3 4 to 7 8 to 10 11 +	2 capsules or ½ tsp per day, in divided doses 3 capsules or ¾ tsp per day, in divided doses 4 capsules or 1 tsp per day, in divided doses 5 capsules or 1¼ tsp per day, in divided doses
VitaSpectrum Multiple for Children with ASD made by *Klaire Labs* *Includes folinic acid, choline, inositol*	2 to 5 6 to 10 11 +	2 capsules per day, in divided doses 4 capsules per day, in divided doses 6 capsules per day, in divided doses
Children's Multi-Vitamin/Mineral Hypoallergenic made by *Kirkman* *Includes folic acid (not folinic acid), CoQ$_{10}$*	2 to 5 6 to 10 11 +	1 capsule per day 2 capsules per day, in divided doses 3 capsules per day, in divided doses
Everyday Multi-Vitamin/Mineral Hypoallergenic made by *Kirkman* *Includes folic acid (not folinic acid), choline, taurine, glutamine*	2 to 5 6 to 10 11 +	1 capsule per day 2 capsules per day, in divided doses 3 capsules per day, in divided doses
Children's Chewable Multi-Vitamin Mineral with Xylitol made by *Kirkman* *Includes folic acid (not folinic acid); CoQ$_{10}$; low calcium; vitamins A, B, C, D, E; biotin*	3 to 5 6 to 10 11 +	½ to 1 wafer per day 2 wafers per day, in divided doses 3 wafers per day, in divided doses
Pure Encapsulations Nutrient 950 made by *Pure Encapsulations* *Includes folinic acid* *Other versions: without iron; without copper and iron; without copper, iron, and iodine; with vitamin K* *For autism, the version without copper is preferred.*	2 to 5 6 to 10 11 +	1 to 2 capsules per day, in divided doses 3 capsules per day, in divided doses 4 capsules per day, in divided doses

BASIC MULTIPLES WITHOUT VITAMINS A AND D	AGE	DOSING WITH MEALS
Everyday Multi-Vitamin/Mineral without Vitamins A & D Hypoallergenic made by *Kirkman* *Includes folic acid (not folinic acid), choline, taurine, glutamine*	2 to 5 6 to 10 11 +	1 capsule per day, emptied in food 2 capsules per day, in divided doses 3 capsules per day, in divided doses

BASIC MULTIPLES WITHOUT VITAMINS A, D, AND B COMPLEX	AGE	DOSING WITH MEALS
Nu-Thera/EveryDay Companion Hypoallergenic made by *Kirkman* *Calcium level is good*	1 to 3 4 to 7 8 to 10 11 +	2 capsules or ⅓ tsp, daily emptied in food 2 capsules or ⅓ tsp, 2 times per day 3 capsules or ½ tsp, 2 times per day 4 capsules or ¾ tsp, 2 times per day

Quick Start: Multivitamins

The dosing instructions above give the goal ranges, and introduction should be "low and slow." Start with half the goal dose and increase to the full dose after three to six days. As you increase, if there are negative symptoms, cut back to the earlier dose that was tolerated. Do not be concerned if your child is unable to take the full dose. Your child should be under the care of a health care practitioner if he or she needs a mutlitple–vitamin that is more therapeutic or needs to exceed the recommended dosage.

■ 1.3 Fuel Stop: The Quick Start Diet—A Healthy Organic Diet

If your child already eats a healthy diet of organic foods or has started on or mastered one of the special diets in this book, congratulations and keep up the good work. If you have not started "cleaning up" your child's diet, you can at any time. There is only the potential for benefits, ranging from better overall health to reduction of many of the neurological and behavioral symptoms.

You can institute a basic healthy diet before, during, or after introducing supplements. The combination of a basic healthy diet and appropriate nutritional supplementation provides a substantial foundation for your journey into treating your child's metabolic, behavioral, developmental, neurological, and/or physical symptoms.

FOOD CATEGORY	UNIT OF MEASURE	AGES 2 TO 5	AGES 6 TO 10	AGES 11 +
Calories		1,200 to 1,400	1,200 to 2,000	1,600 to 2,400
Protein*	Grams	25 to 30	45	60 to 75
Vegetables	Cups	1 to 1.5	2 to 2.5	2 to 3
Fruits	Cups	1 to 1.5	1.5 to 2	1.5 to 2
Grains	Ounce equivalents	3 to 4	5 to 6	6 to 8
Fiber	Grams	10 to 15	15	20 or more
Water	Ounces	32 to 40	40 to 56	56 to 88

* Seafood, poultry, meat, eggs, beans, nuts, seeds, and milk products (as tolerated)

Summary of the Quick Start Diet Recommendations
1. **Include:**
   • Organic, fresh (and fresh frozen) foods
   • Protein at every meal and snack: seafood, poultry, meat, eggs, beans, nuts, seeds, and milk products as tolerated
   • Low-sugar foods for glycemic control
   • Nutrient-dense foods

- Safe, healthy seafood (see the Environmental Working Group, www.ewg.org, and the Environmental Defense Fund, www.edf.org, for recommendations)
- Foods from pastured and grass-fed animals
- Fermented foods (preferably homemade: yogurt, kefir, coconut yogurt, vegetables, fruits, kombucha)
- Homemade bone broths
- Good fats and oils: extra virgin olive oil, avocado, coconut, almond, flax, and butter
- Healthy drinks: clean filtered water, raw vegetable juices, coconut water, coconut milk, almond milk

2. Avoid:
- Pesticides in foods
- Artificial sweeteners, additives, preservatives, coloring, flavors, and MSG
- High-fructose corn syrup (HFCS)
- Sodas (diet and regular)
- Hydrogenated oils/trans fatty acids, (e.g., margarine)
- Homogenized milk products
- Deep-fried foods
- Reaction-provoking foods
- Alcohol (none for children and pregnant women, limited in adults)
- Sugar
- Caffeine
- Craved foods
- Canned foods
- Processed foods
- Refined grains (e.g., bread, pasta, cold cereals, instant hot cereals)

Resources for a healthy diet:
- *Nourishing Traditions* by Sally Fallon
- *Cooking to Heal* by Julie Matthews
- *The Petit Appetit Cookbook* by Lisa Barnes

Quick Start: Diet

CHAPTER 2

Moving Forward: Supplementation Based on Specific Signs and Symptoms

In the previous chapter we discussed the most commonly needed and effective supplements to provide an overall foundation of treatment. This chapter targets more specific physical, behavioral, and developmental symptoms that your child may exhibit.

For each symptom, we will address the following:
· Overview of the symptom
· Main possible nutritional contributing factors
· How to determine which supplement(s) and diet(s) are potentially relevant to your child
· Why that supplement may be beneficial
· What supplements to use and why
· Dosing
· Potential side effects

As with the previous section, please note that doses listed are total daily doses unless otherwise indicated. This means that if a supplement is recommended for more than one symptom, do not exceed the total daily dose for that supplement. For example, if the section on hyperactivity recommends magnesium at a dose of 200 mg/day and the section on anxiety also recommends magnesium at a dose of 200 mg/day, your child's total daily dose should be 200 mg/day, not 400 mg/day. Increasing beyond the total daily dose should be accomplished only under the guidance of a health care practitioner.

■ 2.1 Allergies

Allergies are common in children, including those with behavioral or developmental disorders. The histamine generated from allergies can cause or exacerbate symptoms that interfere with optimal learning and behavior.

Symptoms/signs your child may exhibit
· Runny nose
· Sneezing

- Itchy eyes or nose
- Dark circles under eyes ("allergic shiners")
- Eczema/atopic dermatitis, hives
- Food-induced rash around the mouth
- Food-induced redness around the anus, especially after a bowel movement

Main possible contributing factors
- Environmental triggers (e.g., dust, pollen, grasses, trees)
- Food triggers
- Animal dander

Main helpful supplements
- Quercetin (section A)
- Pantothenic acid/vitamin B$_5$ (section B)
- Vitamin C (section C)

General Information

Children with autism or ADHD may have coexisting allergies. There is sometimes confusion about the distinction between allergies and intolerances and the role of allergies in causing symptoms of these disorders.

Allergies are reactions mediated by specific antibodies called IgE (immunoglobulin E) antibodies. These reactions often occur soon after ingestion or contact with the offending agent and may involve obvious physical symptoms such as hives, rashes, or respiratory symptoms. They do not in and of themselves produce developmental symptoms. However, the histamine generated by these reactions can exacerbate symptoms such as inattention, anxiety, and more.

Food reactions that may result in behavioral or developmental symptoms are best referred to as *sensitivities* or *intolerances* rather than allergies. One type of sensitivity is mediated by a different antibody called IgG (immunoglobulin G). These sensitivity reactions often are more delayed, sometimes up to seventy-two hours after ingestion of the offending food (most commonly casein, gluten, or soy). Although there may be physical symptoms, more commonly the main symptoms are behavioral (e.g., tantrums, inattention, anxiety, etc.). A full discussion of food intolerances is beyond the scope of this book. Please refer to our previous book, *The Kid-Friendly ADHD & Autism Cookbook*, for more detailed information.

These are important distinctions to make as they guide testing decisions. Traditional allergy testing (IgE blood testing, skin testing) does not detect IgG food intolerances or other intolerances. Discuss appropriate testing options with a clinical health care practitioner.

The histamine generated from allergies, however, *can* be problematic and can interfere with brain functioning. Histamine is released from mast cells when the cells are exposed to allergens. Histamine causes symptoms typically associated with allergies such as runny nose, nasal congestion, postnasal drip, itchy eyes or nose, and skin rashes. Some of histamine's negative effects are caused by histamine binding to cells, which then result in these symptoms.

Histamine is also an excitatory neurotransmitter that, when elevated, can exacerbate behavioral symptoms. Individuals who already have elevated neuronal histamine are more sensitive to the behavioral effects of histamine-releasing reactions.

The effect of elevated histamine on behavior may include:
- Inattention
- Irritability
- Anxiety
- Sleep disruption
- Obsessive behavior
- Rigidity

What to Do and How to Do It
There are several treatments for excessive histamine:
1. Removing the triggers for allergies
2. Using antihistamine medications
3. Taking supplements that lower histamine (e.g., quercetin, pantothenic acid, and vitamin C)

Removing environmental triggers requires determining which agents are causing symptoms in your child. Common triggers include dust, mold, pollens, and animal dander. Your child's primary-care physician can be helpful in determining which triggers may be important for your child and ordering specific blood testing or referring to an allergist for additional testing.

Antihistamine medications can be useful in treating physical symptoms of allergies. However, they may be less helpful for the brain-based behavioral symptoms. Most antihistamine medications are directed at blocking the attachment of histamine to tissues, but they do not stop the production of histamine. Blocking the attachment of histamine to tissues in the nose will improve symptoms of runny nose and congestion, and in the skin, may help with itching. But to help with brain symptoms, it is important to lower the production of histamine. Histamine elevations in the brain can contribute to behavioral symptoms as described above.

The three supplements suggested may be taken together. Depending on the individual, any one alone or the combination may be effective.

Section A: Quercetin

Quercetin is a plant flavonol that acts as a mast cell stabilizer. It makes the mast cells harder to burst and therefore results in a smaller release of histamine. If less histamine is released, there is less in the bloodstream and, ultimately, less histamine reaching the brain. Quercetin also has anti-inflammatory and antioxidant effects.

How Do I Dose Quercetin?
Quercetin can be used only during acute allergy symptoms to help resolve them, during those seasons in which your child usually has symptoms, or year-round to help prevent symptoms. Dosing can also be adjusted as needed. A child may be on a lower maintenance dose to prevent allergy symptoms but go to a higher dose temporarily when symptoms flare up.

QUERCETIN TOTAL DAILY GOAL DOSING

AGE	MAINTENANCE DOSE	INCREASE FOR ALLERGIES	TOTAL DAILY DOSE
2 to 5	250 mg	250 mg 2 times per day	500 mg
6 to 10	500 mg	500 mg 2 times per day	1,000 mg
11 +	500 mg	500 mg 2 times per day	1,000 mg

What Side Effects Should I Watch for?
Side effects to quercetin are minimal. High doses taken on an empty stomach can cause discomfort or acid reflux symptoms. It is best taken with a meal. Behavioral side effects are not common, and there are no typical side effects to watch for.

What Else Should I Know?
Quercetin is tasteless. However, the powder is bright yellow. Children who are picky eaters or rigid about their foods may reject a change in food or drink color. Suggestions for hiding quercetin include mixing in:
- Liquid or juice given in an opaque sippy cup
- A similar color juice, such as orange juice
- Peanut butter or chocolate syrup
- Juice and freezing in a homemade ice pop

Quercetin can interact with medications including protecting against negative effects; it can also increase or decrease the effectiveness of certain medications, depending upon the person's biochemical individuality. We strongly recommend that higher doses not be used without the guidance of a health care practitioner. It is safe to take with antihistamine medications. Some children's allergy symptoms are severe enough that they may need treatment both with quercetin and traditional allergy medications.

If your child undergoes skin testing for allergies, antihistamine medications or quercetin will interfere with the skin testing. Ask your allergist how many days before the testing you need to stop quercetin. Quercetin will not interfere with blood testing for allergies.

For children with sleep disruption, antihistamine medications are often recommended for short periods of time to "break the cycle" in the hopes of allowing a regular sleep pattern to return. We would not recommend this approach beyond a few nights. Antihistamines affect REM sleep ("dream sleep"), which is the most restorative part of the sleep cycle, so the sleep your child gets on

Allergies

antihistamines is not good quality sleep. Recent studies through the National Institute of Health are also finding decreased REM sleep in a subset of children with autism. Quercetin can decrease histamine and improve sleep, without a known negative effect on REM sleep.

Section B: Pantothenic Acid

Pantothenic acid (B_5) is a water-soluble B vitamin antioxidant that is essential to all forms of life. It is useful in reducing histamine.

How Do I Dose Pantothenic Acid?

Pantothenic acid (B_5) can be taken regularly at maintenance doses, with increases for allergic reactions. The dose range is wide and has been found safe at doses of 10,000 mg or more per day.

PANTOTHENIC ACID TOTAL DAILY GOAL DOSING

AGE	MAINTENANCE DOSE	INCREASE FOR ALLERGIES	TOTAL DAILY DOSE
2 to 5	100 mg per day	100 to 250 mg per day	250 mg
6 to 10	250 mg per day	250 mg 2 or 3 times per day	750 mg
11 +	500 mg per day	500 mg 2 or 3 times per day	1,000 mg

What Side Effects Should I Watch for?

Side effects from pantothenic acid are minimal. There is no toxic level identified, and no Tolerable Upper Level Intake has been established. Higher doses (over 5,000 mg) can cause loose stools in some individuals.

What Else Should I Know?

Pantothenic acid can be taken along with antihistamine medications. It is synergistic with vitamin C and B vitamins. As with quercetin, it is best to avoid taking pantothenic acid when your child is going to have allergy skin testing.

Section C: Vitamin C

Vitamin C (ascorbic acid) is a water-soluble antioxidant, important in immunity, neurotransmitter function, and well known for antihistamine activity. It prevents histamine release and increases the detoxification of histamine. There is an inverse relationship between vitamin C and histamine. Low vitamin-C serum levels result in high histamine levels.

How Do I Dose Vitamin C?

Vitamin C can be taken regularly at maintenance doses, with increases for allergic reactions. The dose range is wide and has been found safe at doses of 10,000 mg or more.

Vitamin C supplements
- Vitamin C 250-mg Hypoallergenic capsules, made by Kirkman Labs
- Buffered Vitamin C Powder Bio-Max Hypoallergenic: ¼ tsp = 1,100 mg, made by Kirkman Labs
- Vitamin C Ascorbic Acid Ultra-fine Powder: ¼ tsp = 1,000 mg, made by Klaire Labs

VITAMIN C TOTAL DAILY GOAL DOSING

AGE	MAINTENANCE DOSE	INCREASE FOR ALLERGIES	TOTAL DAILY DOSE FROM ALL SOURCES
2 to 5	100 mg per day	100 to 250 mg per day	250 mg
6 to 10	250 mg per day	250 mg 2 or 3 times per day	750 mg
11 +	500 mg per day	500 mg 2 or 3 times per day	1,000 mg

What Side Effects Should I Watch for?

The amount of vitamin C for each individual will vary according to need and the health or illness status at the time. Too much can cause a loose stool or diarrhea. The goal is "bowel tolerance," which is that amount of vitamin C that does not cause loose stools.

Vitamin C is nontoxic because it is water soluble and self-limiting. When there is deficiency, higher need, stress, or illness, the absorption of vitamin C increases, resulting in less effect on the stool. As the need declines, less will be absorbed, increasing the potential for loose stools. Direct prolonged tooth contact with unbuffered ascorbic acid vitamin C can erode enamel. This form is best taken in capsules or mixed in a liquid or smoothie.

What Else Should I Know?

Vitamin C can be taken along with antihistamine medications. It is synergistic with pantothenic acid and B vitamins. As with quercetin and pantothenic acid, it is best to avoid taking vitamin C when your child is having allergy skin testing. Vitamin C is contraindicated in the following conditions. Please consult with a physician or specialist.
- Kidney disease of any kind
- Oxalate kidney stone formation (increases with vitamin C use)
- Hemochromatosis (iron storage disease)
- G6PD deficiency (an inherited disorder affecting red blood cells)

Vitamin C supplements often contain corn. If your child has a food sensitivity to corn, you will need a corn-free version. Vitamin C may also be helpful for supporting the immune system and may be a useful supplement if your child has frequent colds or other illnesses.

Allergies

■ 2.2 Anger, Aggression, and/or Self-Injurious Behavior

Anger and aggression can be coexisting problems in children with ADHD or autism. Children with autism may also demonstrate self-injurious behaviors of varying degrees of severity.

Symptoms/signs your child may exhibit
- Easy frustration
- Temper tantrums
- Aggression toward others
- Self-injurious behaviors such as head banging, picking at skin

Main possible contributing factors
- Unrecognized pain or discomfort
- Magnesium deficiency
- Food intolerances/opioid effect
- Excess glutamate and need for GABA
- High histamine from food or inhalant allergies

DETERMINING WHICH SUPPLEMENTS AND DIET CHANGES MAY BE HELPFUL

IF YOUR CHILD HAS ANGER, AGGRESSION, OR SELF-INJURIOUS BEHAVIOR, AND SOME OF THE FOLLOWING SYMPTOMS	SEE THE APPLICABLE SECTION BELOW	DIETARY AND OTHER RECOMMENDATIONS	OTHER SOURCES FOR INFORMATION
Signs of infections or medical conditions	Section A: Physician Evaluation		
Constipation Sound sensitivity Easy startle Mood swings Sleep disruption Excessive sighing	Section B: Magnesium	Section B: Magnesium Higher intake of magnesium-rich foods	Chapter 4: section 4.8 Magnesium and Calcium
Food cravings for milk casein, gluten, and/or soy In a "fog" or "own world" Bowel problems Unexplained laughing High pain tolerance Poor eye contact Attention problems Language delays	Section C: Elimination of Opioid Food Culprits and Digestive Enzymes	Section C: Elimination of Opioid Food Culprits and Digestive Enzymes Chapter 6: Gluten-Free, Casein-Free, Soy-Free diet (GFCFSF)	Chapter 4: section 4.17 Digestive Enzymes Chapter 6: section 6.1 GFCFSF Diet
Hyperactivity Tics Language delay	Section D: Need for GABA and Vitamin B_6	Section D: Need for GABA and Vitamin B_6 Limit/avoid glutamate (excitotoxins)	Chapter 4: section 4.11 GABA and Theanine and section 4.5 Vitamin B_6
Allergies Runny nose Itchy eyes or nose Allergic shiners Eczema	Section E: Histamine Reduction	Section E: Histamine Reduction	Chapter 2: section 2.1 Allergies

Section A: Physician Evaluation

Before considering dietary or supplement interventions for these symptoms, it is critically important to consider whether your child's behavior is a response to a painful trigger. This is particularly significant if your child is nonverbal or has limited communication abilities and cannot accurately indicate a source of discomfort. Common sources of pain to consider include:

- Ear infection
- Sore throat
- Headache
- Constipation or gas. This can sometimes be missed, as children may be having daily stools but not completely evacuating. An abdominal X-ray can show whether your child is impacted and needs more aggressive treatment to "clean out" the backup.
- Gastroesophageal reflux ("heartburn"). This is often missed. Clues to consider include decrease in appetite, severe resistance to going to sleep (reflux is worse when lying down), night waking, and worsened behavioral symptoms after eating.
- Dental pain (e.g., toothache, abscess)
- Head pain secondary to gluten sensitivity (see section C below)

A thoughtful evaluation by a physician is the most important first step.

Section B: Magnesium

Magnesium has calming effects on the nervous system. When magnesium is deficient, the following symptoms can occur, contributing to anger and self-injurious behaviors:

- Constipation (can contribute to worsened behavior because of physical discomfort as well as inadequate excretion of toxins)
- ADHD symptoms, including hyperactivity and inattention
- Sound or light sensitivity
- Mood dysregulation, depression, anxiety, emotional overreactions
- Irritability, aggression, impulsivity
- Neuromuscular excitability, easy startle, brisk reflexes
- Sleep disruption, nightmares, night terrors

What to Do and How to Do It

Provided here is a brief summary on magnesium. For thorough information and specific guidelines on dosing and side effects, see section 4.8 Magnesium and Calcium.

Magnesium supplements

- Gentle (less laxative) stool effect: chelates, aspartates, glycinates, gluconates, and bisglycinates
- Laxative stool effect: citrates, chlorides, sulfates

Anger

MAGNESIUM TOTAL DAILY GOAL DOSING

AGE	DOSE	FREQUENCY	TOTAL DAILY DOSE FROM ALL SOURCES
2 to 5	100 mg	1 or 2 times per day	200 mg
6 to 10	100 mg	2 or 3 times per day	300 mg
11 +	100 to 150 mg	2 or 3 times per day	450 mg

- Start at one-quarter to one-half of the recommended dose and increase the dose gradually every one to two days.
- Magnesium can cause loose stools or diarrhea.
- Watch for possible side effects and decrease the dose accordingly.
- If symptoms improve at doses lower than the goal, you may not need to continue to increase the dose.
- For higher than recommended doses, consult with a skilled health care practitioner.

Calcium
Calcium intake should be adequate when taking magnesium. Excess magnesium intake can lower calcium, and excess calcium intake can lower magnesium. It is important to have balance. If your child is not getting sufficient calcium from diet, a calcium supplement is indicated.

CALCIUM TOTAL DAILY GOAL DOSING

AGE	DOSE	FREQUENCY	TOTAL DAILY DOSE FROM ALL SOURCES
2 to 5	250 mg	2 times per day	500 mg
6 to 10	250 mg	3 times per day	750 mg
11 +	500 to 600 mg	2 times per day	1,000 to 1,200 mg

Section C: Elimination of Opioid Food Culprits and Digestive Enzymes
An abbreviated discussion of food intolerances in ADHD and autism is available in chapter 4. A full discussion is beyond the scope of this book. Refer to the following resources:
- *The Kid-Friendly ADHD & Autism Cookbook* by the authors
- *Special Diets for Special Kids Volumes 1 and 2 Combined* by Lisa Lewis
- *Cooking to Heal* by Julie Matthews
- The Gluten-Free Casein-Free Diet Intervention—Autism Diet, www.gfcfdiet.com

In short, food proteins, particularly those from milk (casein) and wheat (gluten), may be incompletely digested to peptides and enter the bloodstream from the intestine via an abnormally permeable intestinal lining (referred to as "leaky gut"). These partially digested protein peptides can potentially cross the blood–brain barrier, negatively affecting brain function, including contributing to mood and behavior by several mechanisms:

- Blocking neurotransmitter messages
- Causing opiate-like doping effects from gluten (gliadorphin), milk casein (casomorphin), and soy
- Triggering brain inflammation

The most obvious symptom is a craving for the food opiate sources (gluten, milk products, and soy). Other symptoms include anger, aggression, self-injurious behavior and also hyperactivity, self-stimulatory behaviors, and irritability. Effects may occur within an hour of consumption or be delayed up to seventy-two hours.

What to Do and How to Do It
Provided here is a brief summary of two main treatment strategies for food intolerances and the opiate-like peptide effect.
1. Gluten-free, Casein-free, Soy-free Diet (GFCFSF)—Elimination Trial: the "gold standard" for treatment
   - The most common problem food proteins are gluten, milk casein, and soy. This diet eliminates all three.
   - Your child's body is the best test. Eliminate the food(s) to see whether behavior improves and reintroduce or challenge the body to see whether behavior worsens.
2. Digestive enzyme supplements, including dipeptidyl peptidase-IV (DPP-IV)
   - These supplements help to more efficiently digest gluten, casein, soy and other food proteins, carbohydrates, and fats.
   - They also reduce the opioid load due to insufficient DPP-IV enzyme function; this can also "mimic" the diet.

Digestive Enzyme Supplements
See section 4.17 Digestive Enzymes for detailed information on specific enzyme products and dosing.

Section D: Need for GABA and Vitamin B$_6$

Glutamate is a transmitter with excitatory effects in the brain. Excitatory glutamate converts to the calming neurotransmitter, gamma-aminobutyric acid (GABA). The amount of glutamate can increase in the brain if there is inefficiency in the glutamate decarboxylase enzyme or deficiency of vitamin B$_6$, which is necessary for the enzyme to function.

High glutamate is found in additives such as MSG and aspartame, which are the most problematic sources, and also in processed foods, milk products, grains, peanuts, and meats.

The negative effects of glutamate in the brain are modulated by the calming amino acid and inhibitory neurotransmitter GABA, which may be helpful for treating symptoms such as anger, aggression, self-injurious behaviors and also anxiety, obsessive–compulsive symptoms, perseverative behaviors, irritability, sleep problems, and language delays.

Anger

What to Do and How to Do It
Provided here is a brief summary on GABA. For more information, see section 4.11
GABA and Theanine.
- GABA is best absorbed on an empty stomach, but it may also be taken with food.
- GABA's beneficial effects may affect the dosing of medications used for ADHD, anxiety, and seizures.
- GABA should not be used if the child is already taking a medication that increases or potentially affects GABA, such as benzodiazepines, barbiturates, narcotics, and gabapentin.
- GABA, especially at higher doses, should only be used under the guidance of a health care practitioner.
- Side effects can include lethargy, excitability, and irritability.

GABA TOTAL DAILY GOAL DOSING

AGE	DOSE	FREQUENCY	TOTAL DAILY DOSE FROM ALL SOURCES
2 to 5	25 to 50 mg	2 times per day (breakfast and dinner)	50 to 100 mg
6 to 10	50 to 100 mg	2 times per day (breakfast and dinner)	100 to 200 mg
11 +	250 mg	1 or 2 times per day (breakfast and dinner)	250 to 500 mg

Vitamin B_6
Vitamin B_6 (pyridoxine) and its active form, pyridoxal-5'-phosphate (P5P), are necessary for the enzyme glutamate decarboxylase to convert excitatory glutamate to calming GABA.

What to Do and How to Do It
Some multiple vitamin supplements will have B_6 and/or P5P, which may be sufficient and not require additional supplementation. If they are not being used, supplementation may be necessary. For specifics on B_6 supplementation, see section 4.5 Methylation Nutrients.

Section E: Histamine Reduction
Histamine is a chemical that the body releases in allergic reactions and is usually associated with a runny nose, nasal congestion, postnasal drip, itchy eyes, or nose and skin rashes.

Histamine is also an excitatory neurotransmitter that, when elevated, can increase irritability, frustration, anger, and aggression. Individuals who already have elevated neuronal histamine are more sensitive to the behavioral effects of histamine-releasing reactions. Suspect histamine as contributing to your child's symptoms if behavioral symptoms are worse during allergy seasons.

What to Do and How to Do It
Provided here is a brief summary on histamine. For thorough information and specific guidelines on dosing and side effects, see section 2.1 Allergies. Basic strategies include:

1. Removing the triggers for allergies
   - Inhalants (e.g., grass, trees, pollen, mold, animal danders)
   - Food that causes type I IgE histamine-releasing allergies
2. Using antihistamine medications
3. Taking supplements that reduce histamine release

SUPPLEMENTS THAT REDUCE HISTAMINE RELEASE

SUPPLEMENT	DESCRIPTION	AGE	DAILY DOSE	TOTAL DAILY DOSE FROM ALL SOURCES
Quercetin	Plant flavonol Anti-inflammatory	2 to 5	250 mg 2 times per day	500 mg
		6 to 10	500 mg 2 times per day	1,000 mg
		11 +	500 mg 2 times per day	1,000 mg
Pantothenic acid (vitamin B₅)	Water soluble B vitamin Nontoxic	2 to 5	100 to 250 mg per day	250 mg
		6 to 10	250 mg 2 or 3 times per day	750 mg
		11 +	500 mg 2 times per day	1,000 mg
Vitamin C (ascorbic acid)	Water soluble Nontoxic Excess causes loose stools	2 to 5	100 to 250 mg per day	250 mg
		6 to 10	250 mg 2 or 3 times per day	750 mg
		11 +	500 mg 2 times per day	1,000 mg

- Lower doses can be used for maintenance and reducing allergy potential.
- All three of the supplements may be taken together.
- Antihistamine supplements should not be taken when being skin tested for allergies.

■ 2.3 *Anxiety, Perseverations, Obsessive– Compulsive Symptoms, and Repetitive Behaviors*

Anxiety and the behaviors that may accompany anxiety are common coexisting problems in many children with ADHD and autism. Children with autism are more likely to have obsessions, perseverative or "stuck" behaviors, and repetitive or stereotyped body movements.

Symptoms/signs your child may exhibit
- Anxiety or fears
- Rituals such as lining up objects, needing to touch things symmetrically or do things in a certain order or in a certain way
- Perseverations or obsessions with certain toys, videos, movies, or topics
- Collecting or grouping certain toys or objects
- Hand flapping, finger flicking, toe walking, body rocking

Main possible nutritional contributing factors
- Magnesium deficiency
- Need for taurine
- Low serotonin
- Excess glutamate and need for gamma-aminobutyric acid (GABA)
- Histamine from allergies

DETERMINING WHICH SUPPLEMENTS AND DIET CHANGES MAY BE HELPFUL

IF YOUR CHILD HAS ANXIETY AND SOME OF THE FOLLOWING SYMPTOMS	SEE THE APPLICABLE SECTION BELOW	DIETARY AND OTHER RECOMMENDATIONS	OTHER SOURCES FOR INFORMATION
Constipation Sound sensitivity Easy startle Mood swings Sleep disruption Excessive sighing	Section A: Magnesium and Taurine	Higher intake of magnesium-rich foods, e.g., vegetables, beans, nuts, seeds, fruits	Chapter 4: section 4.8 Magnesium and Calcium and section 4.12 Taurine
Obsessive-compulsive behaviors Perseverations Depressed mood Sleep disorder	Section B: Serotonin Support	Starches at bedtime	
Hyperactivity Tics Language delay	Section C: High Glutamate and Need for GABA and Vitamin B$_6$	Limit/avoid glutamate (excitotoxins), e.g., MSG, milk products, gluten, aspartame	Chapter 4: section 4.11 GABA and Theanine and section 4.5 Vitamin B$_6$
Allergy symptoms: Dark circles under the eyes (allergic shiners) Nasal congestion Runny nose Itchy eyes or nose Eczema Asthma Dermatographia (raised red marks in areas that are scratched)	Section D: Histamine Reduction	Avoidance of Type I, IGE-mediated allergens: Inhalants (grasses, trees, pollen, molds) Reaction-provoking foods	Chapter 2: section 2.1 Allergies

Section A: Magnesium and Taurine

Magnesium has calming effects on the nervous system. Low magnesium levels result in neuromuscular excitability. A deficiency can increase anxiety, obsessive–compulsive behaviors, perseverations, and repetitive behaviors. Magnesium is a common nutritional deficiency in both children with ADHD or autism and the general population.

What to Do and How to Do It
Provided here is a brief summary on magnesium. For thorough information and specific guidelines on dosing and side effects, see chapter 4.
    Magnesium supplements:
- Gentle (less laxative) stool effect: chelates, aspartates, glycinates, gluconates, and bisglycinates
- Laxative stool effect: citrates, chlorides, sulfates

MAGNESIUM TOTAL DAILY GOAL DOSING

AGE	DOSE	FREQUENCY	TOTAL DAILY DOSE FROM ALL SOURCES
2 to 5	100 mg	1 or 2 times per day	200 mg
6 to 10	100 mg	2 or 3 times per day	300 mg
11 +	100 to 150 mg	2 or 3 times per day	450 mg

- Start at one-quarter to one-half of the recommended dose and increase the dose gradually every one to two days.
- Magnesium can cause loose stools or diarrhea (which then can deplete magnesium).
- Watch for possible side effects and decrease the dose accordingly.
- If symptoms improve at lower than the goal dose, you may not need to continue to increase the dose.
- For higher-than-recommended doses, consult with a skilled health care practitioner.

Taurine is a sulfur-bearing amino acid that improves magnesium cellular uptake and utilization. It is also a calming amino acid that supports GABA, an inhibitory neurotransmitter. If your child has an autism disorder, only use taurine under the guidance of a health care practitioner. A subset of children with autism have metabolic disorders, some of which may render them intolerant to specific amino acids, including taurine.

Starting with low doses will reveal any negative responses, which should resolve upon cessation. Blood and urine amino acid testing and a metabolic workup will be helpful in guiding the safe use of taurine.

TAURINE TOTAL DAILY GOAL DOSING

AGE	DOSE	FREQUENCY	TOTAL DAILY DOSE FROM ALL SOURCES
2 to 5	150 mg	1 or 2 times per day	300 mg
6 to 10	150 mg	2 times per day	300 mg
11 +	250 mg	2 times per day	500 mg

- Start at half of the lowest recommended dose and increase as tolerated.
- Watch for possible side effects and decrease the dose accordingly.
- If symptoms improve at doses lower than the goal, you may not need to continue to increase the dose.

Calcium

Calcium intake should be adequate when taking magnesium. Excess magnesium intake can lower calcium, and excess calcium intake can lower magnesium. It is important to have balance. If your child is not getting sufficient calcium from diet, a calcium supplement is indicated.

Anxiety

CALCIUM TOTAL DAILY GOAL DOSING

AGE	DOSE	FREQUENCY	TOTAL DAILY DOSE FROM ALL SOURCES
2 to 5	250 mg	2 times a day	500 mg
6 to 10	250 mg	3 times a day	750 mg
11 +	500 to 600 mg	2 times a day	1,000 to 1,200 mg

Section B: Serotonin Support

Serotonin is an important transmitter in the brain that affects mood, emotions, behavior, appetite, cognition, and sleep. The amino acid tryptophan converts to 5-HTP (5-Hydroxytryptophan), which then converts to serotonin; serotonin then converts to melatonin. Magnesium, vitamin B_3 (niacinamide), and vitamin B_6 (pyridoxine) are important in serotonin metabolism. Low levels of serotonin can result in anxiety, depression, mood disorders, irritability, obsessive–compulsive symptoms, repetitive movements, and sleep disorders.

What to Do and How to Do It

There are three main ways to raise serotonin:
1. Medications such as Selective Serotonin Reuptake Inhibitors (SSRIs):
   - SSRIs and 5-HTP raise serotonin levels in the brain but by different mechanisms.
   - Serotonin is released by neurons (nerve cells) in the brain and taken back up by these cells in order to be reused.
   - SSRIs block this uptake so that the serotonin effect is prolonged.
   - SSRIs must be prescribed and monitored by a physician.
2. Direct nutritional support of the serotonin pathway via tryptophan and 5-HTP:
   - 5-HTP supplementation produces more serotonin directly as compared to L-tryptophan.
   - 5-HTP should be used only under the care of a knowledgeable health care practitioner.
   - The use of tryptophan and/or 5-HTP is not recommended when taking an SSRI medication because there is the risk for excessive serotonin.
   - Opposite reactions such as hyperactivity or insomnia, and/or manic symptoms may occur.
3. Serotonin nutrient cofactor supplementation:
   - Magnesium, zinc, iron, methylation support (B_6, B_{12}, folinic acid), and vitamin B_3

These nutrients are essential to optimal serotonin metabolism. Use of a good multivitamin is a start for providing these nutrient cofactors. More specific supplement adjustment is best done with guidance by a skilled health care practitioner (physician or nutritionist).

Section C: High Glutamate and Need for GABA and Vitamin B₆

Glutamate is a transmitter with excitatory effects in the brain. Excitatory glutamate converts to the calming neurotransmitter, GABA. Glutamate can increase in the brain if there is inefficiency in the glutamate decarboxylase enzyme or deficiency of vitamin B_6, which is necessary for the enzyme to function.

High glutamate is found in additives such as MSG and aspartame, which are the most problematic sources, and also in processed foods, milk products, grains, peanuts, and meats.

The negative effects of glutamate in the brain are modulated by the calming amino acid and inhibitory neurotransmitter, GABA, which may be helpful for treating symptoms such as anxiety and also anger, aggression, obsessive–compulsive symptoms, perseverative behaviors, irritability, sleep problems, and language delays.

What to Do and How to Do It
Provided here is a brief summary on GABA. For more thorough information, see section 4.11 GABA and Theanine.

GABA supplements:
- GABA is best absorbed on an empty stomach, but may be taken with food.
- GABA's beneficial effects may affect dosing of medications used for ADHD, anxiety, and seizures. Do not add GABA without discussing it first with your child's prescribing physician.
- GABA should not be used if the child is already taking a medication that increases or potentially affects GABA, such as benzodiazepines, barbiturates, narcotics, and gabapentin.
- GABA, especially at higher doses, should only be used under the guidance of a health care practitioner.
- Side effects can include lethargy, excitability, or irritability.

GABA TOTAL DAILY GOAL DOSING

AGE	DOSE	FREQUENCY	TOTAL DAILY DOSE FROM ALL SOURCES
2 to 5	25 to 50 mg	2 times per day (breakfast and dinner)	50 to 100 mg
6 to 10	50 to 100 mg	2 times per day (breakfast and dinner)	100 to 200 mg
11 +	250 mg	1 or 2 times per day (breakfast and dinner)	250 to 500 mg

Vitamin B₆
Vitamin B_6 (pyridoxine) and its active form, pyridoxal-5′-phosphate (P5P), are necessary for the enzyme glutamate decarboxylase to convert excitatory glutamate to calming GABA.

What to Do and How to Do It
Some multiple vitamin supplements will have B_6 and/or P5P, which may be sufficient and not require additional supplementation. If they are not being used, supplementation may be necessary. For specifics on B_6 supplementation, see section 4.5 Methylation Nutrients.

Section D: Histamine Reduction

Histamine is a chemical released in allergic conditions and is usually associated with a runny nose, nasal congestion, postnasal drip, itchy eyes or nose, and skin rashes.

Histamine is also an excitatory neurotransmitter that, when elevated, can increase anxiety. Individuals who already have elevated neuronal histamine are more sensitive to the behavioral effects of histamine-releasing reactions. Suspect histamine as contributing to your child's symptoms if behavioral symptoms are worse during allergy seasons.

When anxiety interferes with sleep and allergies are an issue, antihistamine medications can be used short term to reduce the sleep disruption from histamine. However, they can also interfere with REM sleep, the most restorative part of the sleep cycle. The antihistamine nutrients (quercetin, pantothenic acid, and vitamin C) do not interfere with the sleep cycle.

What to Do and How to Do It
Provided here is a brief summary on histamine. For thorough information and specific guidelines on dosing and side effects, see section 2.1 Allergies. Basic strategies include:
1. Removing the triggers for allergies
   - Inhalants (e.g., grass, trees, pollen, mold, animal danders)
   - Food that causes type I IgE histamine-releasing allergies
2. Using antihistamine medications
3. Taking supplements that reduce histamine release

SUPPLEMENTS THAT REDUCE HISTAMINE RELEASE

SUPPLEMENT	DESCRIPTION	AGE	DAILY DOSE	TOTAL DAILY DOSE FROM ALL SOURCES
Quercetin	Plant flavonol Anti-inflammatory	2 to 5	250 mg 2 times per day	500 mg
		6 to 10	500 mg 2 times per day	1,000 mg
		11 +	500 mg 2 times per day	1,000 mg
Pantothenic acid (vitamin B_5)	Water soluble B vitamin Nontoxic	2 to 5	100 to 250 mg per day	250 mg
		6 to 10	250 mg 2 or 3 times per day	750 mg
		11 +	500 mg 2 times per day	1,000 mg
Vitamin C (ascorbic acid)	Water soluble Nontoxic Excess causes loose stools	2 to 5	100 to 250 mg per day	250 mg
		6 to 10	250 mg 2 or 3 times per day	750 mg
		11 +	500 mg 2 times per day	1,000 mg

- Lower doses can be used for maintenance and reducing allergy potential.
- All three of the supplements may be taken together and also with antihistamine medications.
- "Antihistamine" supplements should not be taken when being skin tested for allergies.

■ *2.4 Attention and Focus Problems*

Inattention is a cardinal symptom of ADHD and is very common in children with autism. Inattention clearly interferes with academic learning but has social consequences as well.

Symptoms/signs your child may exhibit

- Short attention span
- Daydreaming
- "In a fog" or appearing "in his or her own world"
- Distractibility
- Difficulty completing tasks
- Not appearing to listen/hear when spoken to

Main possible contributing factors

- Deficiencies in:
  - — Omega-3 fatty acids
  - — Zinc
  - — Vitamin D
  - — Iron
  - — B_{12} and folinic acid
- Food intolerances, including opiate-like peptides (e.g., from casein, gluten, soy)
- Toxins from yeast
- Excess glutamate and need for gamma-aminobutyric acid (GABA)
- Excess histamine (e.g., from allergies)
- Low blood sugar because of a diet that's low in protein and/or high in refined carbohydrates

DETERMINING WHICH SUPPLEMENTS AND DIET CHANGES MAY BE HELPFUL

IF YOUR CHILD HAS INATTENTION AND SOME OF THE FOLLOWING SYMPTOMS	SEE THE APPLICABLE SECTION BELOW	DIETARY AND OTHER RECOMMENDATIONS	OTHER SOURCES OF INFORMATION
Cracking, peeling, chipping nails Language delays Vision dysfunction Excessive thirst Hard earwax	Section A: Essential Omega-3 Fatty Acids		Chapter 4: section 4.15 Essential Omega-3 Fatty Acids

IF YOUR CHILD HAS INATTENTION AND SOME OF THE FOLLOWING SYMPTOMS	SEE THE APPLICABLE SECTION BELOW	DIETARY AND OTHER RECOMMENDATIONS	OTHER SOURCES OF INFORMATION
Picky appetite White lines on nails Frequent illness Eczema/dermatitis Language delays Developmental delays Growth delays Sensory sensitivities Inattention Highly refined "white" diet	Section B: Zinc	Good protein intake Low intake of refined carbohydrates	Chapter 4: section 4.9 Zinc
Scaly, cracked "ring around the mouth" Profuse sweating Delayed tooth eruption Bowing legs Bulging forehead "Knobby" knees or ankles Developmental delays	Section C: Vitamin D	Sun exposure, if tolerated	Chapter 4: section 4.2 Vitamin D
Fatigue Decreased energy Pale skin Pallor inside lower eyelid Nail bed pallor upon pressure Dizzy upon standing Craving for chewing ice	Section D: Iron	Red meat, chicken, seafood, beans, nuts, seeds	
Fatigue Language delays Cognitive problems Learning delay Language delay Poor eye contact	Section E: Vitamin B$_6$, Methyl B$_{12}$, and Folinic Acid		Chapter 4: section 4.5 Methylation Nutrients: B$_{12}$, Folinic Acid, B$_6$, DMG, and TMG
Food cravings for milk casein and/or gluten and/or soy In a "fog" or "own world" Bowel problems Unexplained laughing High pain tolerance Poor eye contact Mood problems Language delays	Section F: Food Intolerances and Elimination of Opioid Food Culprits Digestive enzymes	Section F: Food Intolerances and Elimination of Opioid Food Culprits Gluten-Free, Casein-Free, Soy-Free (GFCFSF) diet	Chapter 4: section 4.17 Digestive Enzymes Chapter 6: section 6.1 GFCFSF Diet
Recurrent antibiotic use Coated tongue Thrush Diaper rashes Redness around the anus	Section G: Treating Intestinal Yeast Overgrowth Probiotics Biotin Antifungal herbs	Section G: Treating Intestinal Yeast Overgrowth Antifungal medications Anti-yeast diet	Chapter 2: section 2.18 Yeast Overgrowth Chapter 4: section 4.16 Probiotics and section 4.6 Biotin Chapter 6: section 6.4 Anti-Yeast/Anti-*Candida* Diet

IF YOUR CHILD HAS INATTENTION AND SOME OF THE FOLLOWING SYMPTOMS	SEE THE APPLICABLE SECTION BELOW	DIETARY AND OTHER RECOMMENDATIONS	OTHER SOURCES OF INFORMATION
Tics Hyperactivity Language delay	Section H: High Glutamate and Need for GABA and Vitamin B_6	Section H: High Glutamate and Need for GABA and Vitamin B_6 Limit/avoid glutamate (excitotoxins)	Chapter 4: section 4.11 GABA and Theanine and section 4.5 B_6
Runny nose, cough, itchy eyes Eczema Asthma Dark circles under eyes	Section I: Histamine Reduction	Avoidance of allergy-causing foods	Chapter 2: section 2.1 Allergies

Attention

Section A: Essential Omega-3 Fatty Acids

The essential omega-3 fatty acids are eicosapentaenoic acid (EPA) and docosahexaenoic acid (DHA). Almost 60 percent of the brain is composed of fat, with DHA being the primary structural component of the human brain and retina. DHA also affects focus and attention.

What to Do and How to Do It

Provided here is a brief summary on omega-3 fatty acids. For thorough information and specific guidelines on supplement brands, dosing, and side effects, see section 4.15 Essential Omega-3 Fatty Acids.

The best food sources of omega-3 fatty acids are seafood. Those highest in mercury, PCBs, and other toxins include tomalley (crab mustard), farmed fish, trout, imported shrimp, and the large "steak" fish such as tuna, bluefish, swordfish, and shark. The safest choices include anchovies, sardines, domestic shrimp, rockfish, and tilapia. For details, see the Environmental Working Group website, www.ewg.org, and the Environmental Defense Fund website, www.edf.org.

Omega-3 supplements
- For focus and attention issues, we recommend that DHA amount be equal to or greater than the EPA.
- Use only direct alpha-linollenic acid (ALA) source EPA and DHA, which is more efficient than flaxseed-source.
- Use toxin-free supplements: pharmaceutical grade or molecular distillation to remove toxins.

Types of high DHA omega-3 supplements available in capsules, liquids, and chewables
- Cod liver oil (contains varying amounts of vitamins A and D)
- Fish oils with increased DHA to EPA ratio
- Vegetarian algae-source DHA

The following supplements have substantial levels of DHA:
- Barleans Omega Swirl
- Omega Cure (unflavored)

- Nordic Naturals ProOmega or Ultimate Omega
- Carlson Norwegian Cod Liver Oil with A and D$_3$
- Genestra Super DHA Liquid
- Nordic Naturals Baby's DHA (and EPA)
- Neuromins DHA caps (algae source DHA)
- Nordic Naturals ProDHA 1,000 soft gels

EPA AND DHA TOTAL DAILY GOAL DOSING

AGE	EPA	DHA	FREQUENCY
2 to 5	200 to 400 mg	200 to 400 mg	Daily with food
6 to 10	500 to 650 mg	400 to 500 mg	Daily with food
11 +	500 to 800 mg	500 to 650 mg	Daily with food

- Though DHA is preferred for assisting in attention, focus, eye contact, and communication, EPA is also important and should be included.
- Higher-than-recommended doses of omega-3 fatty acids should only be given under the guidance of a skilled health care practitioner.

For vitamin A content, make sure that the total from cod liver oil, the multiple vitamin–mineral supplement, and additional vitamin A does not exceed the dosing guidelines found in section 4.1 Vitamin A and Beta-Carotene.

Section B: Zinc

Zinc deficiency can result in poor attention and other problems that can contribute to inattention: poor eye contact, developmental delays, sensory deficits, vision dysfunction, auditory processing problems, communication delays, and poor glucose control. Other symptoms of zinc deficiency include poor muscle endurance, growth delays, and picky appetite.

Zinc deficiency can stem from poor intake, higher needs, and/or depletion by a glycemic diet, medications, or toxins. Zinc is part of the insulin molecule and depleted by diets that are glycemic (raise blood sugar quickly). Low zinc levels lead to poor appetite for healthy foods and an increased appetite for the "quick fix" foods (e.g., pasta, breads, crackers, pretzels, sweets, sodas, and juices).

What to Do and How to Do It

Provided here is a brief summary on zinc. For thorough information and specific guidelines on dosing and side effects, see section 4.9 Zinc.

Zinc supplements
- Well tolerated: gluconates, chelates, citrates, acetates, picolinates, chlorides, and bisglycinates
- Strong taste, needs disguising: sulfates

ZINC TOTAL DAILY GOAL DOSING

AGE	DOSE	FREQUENCY	TOTAL DAILY DOSE FROM ALL SOURCES
2 to 5	5 to 10 mg	1 or 2 times per day	10 to 20 mg
6 to 10	10 mg	2 times per day	20 mg
11 +	10 to 15 mg	2 times per day	20 to 30 mg

For optimal oral absorption, an empty stomach is best, but it may not be feasible if nausea occurs. Large doses can cause gastric discomfort, nausea, and inhibit the digestive enzyme DPP-IV (digests opioids from gluten and casein). In addition:

- Avoid or limit giving oral zinc at the same time as interfering nutrients such as calcium, iron, folate, and phosphorylated nutrients (R5P, P5P, phosphatidylcholine); this may not always be feasible.
- Consider using a topical zinc lotion by Kirkman Labs (22 mg of zinc per scoop). Apply to muscle areas in which absorption is highest: shoulders, back, or calves. If you are using other topical supplements, do not mix the lotions together.
- Zinc excess can lower copper levels. Copper levels need to be maintained.
- Use the Zinc Tally Taste Test on page 213 for evaluating progress.
- Higher doses may be required because of poor absorption, antacid use, the presence of toxic metals in the body, or lab findings. This should be accomplished with a skilled health care practitioner.

Diet Balanced in Protein with Low-Glycemic Refined Carbohydrates

Zinc deficiency can occur because of a diet that's low in good protein and high in refined, glycemic carbohydrates (foods that raise blood sugar). This "white" diet includes bread, pasta, crackers, cheese, milk products, and low intake of vegetables. Glycemic diets trigger increased production of insulin, which has zinc as part of the molecular structure. The high demand for insulin depletes zinc (and also chromium), leading to poor glucose control.

Zinc is responsible for the utilization, digestion, and absorption of amino acids from protein intake. Even if protein intake is excellent, if zinc is deficient, then the amino acids from protein are not utilized well by the body. This can result in low blood sugar levels leading to poor attention and also fatigue and poor muscle endurance.

What to Do and How to Do It

A diet that stabilizes blood glucose and leads to improved focus and attention includes the following:

- Good protein intake (at every meal and snack) from seafood, poultry, meat, eggs, beans, nuts, seeds, and milk products (if tolerated).
- High fiber from vegetables, beans, nuts, seeds, fruits, and cooked whole-grain cereals
- Avoidance of all artificial sweeteners because they disrupt glucose control and increase hunger

Attention

- Avoidance of glycemic sugars, juices, dried fruits, sodas, and refined flour grains (breads, pastas, crackers, pretzels, crackers, and cookies)

Section C: Vitamin D

Vitamin D deficiency is very common. It is important for brain development and cognition. Deficiencies affect attention, focus, development, communication, immunity, and skin health. Risk factors for deficiency of vitamin D include inadequate sun exposure (or use of sunblock), darker skin pigmentation, obesity, breast feeding, low dietary intake, and fat malabsorption.

What to Do and How to Do It

Provided here is a brief summary on vitamin D. See section 4.2 for more information on functions, products, dosing, and side effects.

Vitamin D supplements
- Vitamin D_3 is available in capsules, tablets, and liquids.
- The micellized version of vitamin D_3 is a water-soluble form of vitamin D that is well absorbed and especially useful in conditions where absorption is poor.
- Vitamin D_3 (cholecalciferol) is the best form to use for supplementation.
- Vitamin D_2 (ergocalciferol) converts to vitamin D_3 and is less effective long term.
- The oil and micellized forms are preferred over the dry forms.

VITAMIN D TOTAL DAILY GOAL DOSING

AGE	DOSE	FREQUENCY
2 to 5	400 to 600 IU	Daily
6 to 10	600 to 800 IU	Daily
11 +	800 to 2,000 IU	Daily

- The total daily dose includes all sources such as from cod liver oil and multiple vitamins.
- Do blood testing (25-hydroxy vitamin D) to guide dosing. The optimal goal level is 60 to 80 ng/ml.
- Adequate vitamin A intake must be maintained. See section 4.1 for vitamin A dosing.
- Higher doses of vitamins D and A should be accomplished with the help of a health care practitioner.

Section D: Iron

Iron-deficiency anemia contributes to decreased attention, arousal, and social responsiveness, most often observed in ADHD. The symptoms occur because iron is responsible for oxygen delivery to the tissues. Muscle function, tone, and endurance are iron-dependent. Iron is one of the important cofactors in carnitine production (see section E, which follows). Iron (as well as tetrahydrofolate and tyrosine) is necessary for the synthesis of dopamine, the neurotransmitter most involved in attention. Iron deficiency is found in individuals with ADHD and autism.

Body stores of iron as shown by low ferritin levels on blood testing decline first, prior to serum iron declining. These deficits occur before the complete blood count indicates anemia. For this reason, inattention, poor endurance, lethargy, or fatigue may show up before the complete blood count reveals there is a problem.

What to Do and How to Do It

Provided here is a brief summary on iron. Signs of iron deficiency are listed in the table on page 50. Iron should never be given without blood testing to document whether your child has a need for iron. If blood levels of iron are too high or there is a metabolic disorder in which iron accumulates in the tissues, iron supplementation can be damaging and even toxic. Consider these tests to determine levels: complete blood count, serum iron, TIBC, percent saturation, and serum ferritin (a measure of iron stores). When taking iron, routine follow-up blood testing is critical.

Iron dietary sources
- The richest and best-absorbed iron (heme) is found in meats, especially liver.
- Plant sources of iron (nonheme) are less well absorbed (beans, nuts, seeds, and spinach).

Iron supplements:
- All forms of iron supplements can darken the stool (depending upon the dose).
- Iron supplements can cause constipation, especially the sulfate forms.
- Forms that are well tolerated by the digestive tract are ferrous fumarate, gluconate, bisglycinate, and chelates.

IRON TOTAL DAILY GOAL DOSING

AGE	DOSE	FREQUENCY	TOTAL DAILY DOSE FROM ALL SOURCES
2 to 5	7 to 10 mg	Daily	7 to 10 mg
6 to 10	10 mg	Daily	10 mg
11 +	8 to 10 mg	Daily	8 to 10 mg

- We strongly recommend that you do not give iron for the treatment of inattention without consulting with a physician and having appropriate blood testing. Doses based on blood tests may be higher than those indicated in the chart.
- Iron is best not taken at the same time as calcium, zinc, phosphorus, fiber, and vitamin E. The main side effect of treatment with iron is constipation, which can be resolved by avoiding sulfate forms of iron and by adding magnesium and/or vitamin C. See the section on constipation on page 71.

Attention

Section E: Vitamin B_6, Methyl B_{12}, and Folinic Acid

Vitamins B_6, B_{12}, and folinic acid are water-soluble essential nutrients for brain and nerve development and function. They are also critical participants in methylation, a process essential for regulating DNA synthesis and enzymes, building neurotransmitters, synchronizing neuron firing, and creating cellular energy. These functions profoundly affect cognition, focus, attention, and language. These vitamins are among the most common nutrients helpful to children with ADHD and autism.

What to Do and How to Do It

Provided here is a brief summary on vitamins B_6, B_{12}, and folinic acid. For thorough information and specific guidelines on dosing and side effects, see section 4.5 Methylation Nutrients.

Testing for B_6, B_{12}, and folinic acid should be accomplished by a skilled health care practitioner. Serum levels of these vitamins are not sensitive markers for deficiency and do not decline until extreme late stages of deficiency. There are specialized metabolite tests that are more specific for functional status (kynurenic acid for B_6, methylmalonic acid for B_{12}, and formiminoglutamic acid for folate).

Multiple vitamin and B complex supplements may or may not have sufficient levels of these B vitamins. Added doses may be required.

Vitamin B_6
- Pyridoxal-5′-phosphate (P5P) is the active cofactor form.
- B_6 is more effective if taken with magnesium.
- If sulfation is defective, as is the case with phenol sensitivities/intolerances, avoid the P5P form of B_6.
- Absorption can be hindered by antacids.
- Vitamin B_6 and P5P should be taken daily with food before noon.

VITAMIN B_6 AND P5P TOTAL DAILY GOAL DOSING

	AGE	TOTAL DAILY DOSE FROM ALL SOURCES
Vitamin B_6 (pyridoxine)	2 to 5	10 to 15 mg
	6 to 10	20 to 30 mg
	11 +	50 mg
P5P (pyridoxal-5′-phosphate)	2 to 5	5 mg
	6 to 10	10 mg
	11 +	15 mg

Vitamin B_{12}
- Methylcobalamin and hydroxocobalamin are active forms that have excellent bioavailability.
- Poor absorption and/or the use of antacids can cause B_{12} deficiency.
- Sublingual forms may be preferred (they bypass the stomach and small intestine).
- Absorption can be hindered by antacids.
- Methyl B_{12} should be taken daily with food before noon.

METHYL B$_{12}$ TOTAL DAILY GOAL DOSING

AGE	TOTAL DAILY DOSE FROM ALL SOURCES
2 to 5	50 to 100 mcg
6 to 10	100 to 500 mcg
11 +	500 to 1000 mcg

Folinic acid
- Folinic acid is one of the preferred folate forms noted for its excellent bioavailability.
- Folic acid is least effective and best avoided.
- Absorption can be hindered by antacids, antiseizure medications, and tetracycline.
- Folinic acid should be taken daily with or without food.

FOLINIC ACID TOTAL DAILY GOAL DOSING

AGE	TOTAL DAILY DOSE FROM ALL SOURCES
2 to 5	100 mcg
6 to 10	200 mcg
11 +	400 mcg

- All supplements come in liquid, capsule, and tablet forms. Refer to section 4.5 Methylation Nutrients for additional information.
- Side effects can include increased activity, anxiety, and stimming (repeated self-stimulatory behaviors). These are more likely to occur in those children who are overmethylated. If these symptoms occur, stop the supplement and discuss with your health care practitioner.
- Folinic acid can mask the symptoms of pernicious anemia due to B$_{12}$ deficiency. This can be avoided through appropriate testing and pairing folinic acid with vitamin B$_{12}$ supplementation.

Section F: Food Intolerances and Elimination of Opioid Food Culprits

Food intolerances can contribute significantly to inattention and focus problems. A full discussion of food intolerances is beyond the scope of this book. More information and resources are available in section 4.17 Digestive Enzymes and section 6.1 Gluten-Free Casein-Free Soy-Free Diet.

In short, food proteins, particularly those from milk (casein) and wheat (gluten), may be incompletely digested to peptides and may enter the bloodstream from the intestine via an abnormally permeable intestinal lining (referred to as "leaky gut"). These partially digested protein peptides can potentially cross the blood–brain barrier, negatively affecting brain function, including contributing to mood, attention, and behavior by several mechanisms:
- Blocking neurotransmitter messages
- Creating opiate-like doping effects from gluten (gliadorphin), milk casein

Attention

(casomorphin), and soy
• Triggering brain inflammation

The most obvious symptom is a craving for the food opiate sources (gluten, milk products, and soy). In addition to inattention and focus problems, other symptoms can include language delays, poor eye contact, irritability, and increased activity and self-stimulatory behaviors. Effects may occur within an hour of consumption or be delayed up to seventy-two hours.

What to Do and How to Do It
Provided here is a brief summary of two main treatment strategies for food intolerances and the opioid effect.
1. Gluten-Free Casein-Free Soy-Free Diet—Elimination Trial: the "gold standard" for treatment
   • The most common problem food proteins are gluten, milk casein, and soy.
   • Your child's body is the best test. Eliminate the food(s) to see whether behavior improves and reintroduce or challenge the body to see whether behavior worsens.
2. Digestive enzymes, including dipeptidyl peptidase-IV (DPP-IV)
   • More efficiently digest gluten, casein, soy, and other food proteins, carbohydrates, and fats.
   • Reduce the opioid load due to insufficient DPP-IV enzyme function; this can also "mimic" the diet.

Digestive Enzyme Supplements
See section 4.17 Digestive Enzymes for detailed information on specific enzyme products and dosing.

Section G: Treating Intestinal Yeast Overgrowth
Yeast organisms are normal residents of the intestinal tract. Contrary to popular understanding, problematic yeast overgrowth is common in children with a variety of digestive, behavioral, and developmental issues. Treatment may result in notable improvement in a subset of children.

Yeast overgrowth in the intestinal tract can result from inadequate beneficial bacteria because of antibiotic or steroid use, high sugar intake, and/or poor diet, including inadequate fiber. Physical symptoms can include diaper rashes, oral thrush, skin conditions, intestinal inflammation, and abnormal stools. If yeast toxins are absorbed into the bloodstream through an abnormally permeable intestinal lining, behavioral symptoms such as inattention, anxiety, irritability, and silliness or unexplained laughing can occur.

What to Do and How to Do It
Provided here is a brief summary on treatments for yeast overgrowth. For thorough information and more specific guidelines, see section 2.18 Yeast Overgrowth, section 4.16 Probiotics, and section 4.6 Biotin.

Main beneficial treatments:
- Probiotics (beneficial bacteria)
- Biotin
- Antifungal (anti-yeast) medications or herbs
- Anti-yeast diet (anti-*Candida* diet)

Probiotics
Probiotics are beneficial live microorganisms called the microbiome, found throughout the body, including in the intestinal tract. There are more than 100 trillion beneficial bacteria in the body with 500 to 1,000 different species (forty to fifty of which are main species) in the human gut. They maintain healthy flora, prevent overgrowth of harmful pathogens and yeast, and produce healthy nutrients. For a complete listing of probiotic benefits, specific products, and dosing guidelines, see section 2.18 Yeast Overgrowth and section 4.16 Probiotics.

Biotin
Biotin is a water-soluble B vitamin manufactured in the human digestive tract by healthy flora. Antibiotics depress biotin production, which leads to yeast/fungal overgrowth. Biotin helps keep yeast in a less invasive form, which makes it easier to eradicate. Biotin is one of the safest supplements. It has no toxicity at any level. See section 4.6 The Helper B, Biotin, for more information and dosing guidelines.

Antifungal Medications or Herbs
Probiotics help provide beneficial bacteria to the intestinal tract but do not directly kill yeast. To bring yeast levels back down to normal levels, antifungal medications or herbs are used. Probiotics then help maintain good bacterial balance to help prevent yeast overgrowth from recurring.

Antifungal treatments may include herbs or prescription medications. Depending on the amount of yeast present, intestinal symptoms and behavioral side effects from treatment may be significant. Known as "yeast die-off" symptoms, these may include irritability, behavioral regression, and flu-like symptoms. Because of the potential for significant side effects, antifungal treatment should be guided by a health care practitioner based on your child's history and, where possible, specific testing for yeast. See section 2.18, Yeast Overgrowths, for additional treatment information.

Possible yeast treatments include:
- Medications (e.g., Nystatin, Diflucan)
- Herbs (e.g., olive leaf extract, barberry, goldenseal, neem, grapefruit seed extract, pau d'arco, allicin/garlic, caprylic acid, and oregano oil)

Anti-Yeast Diet
The anti-yeast diet avoids foods that "feed" yeast including sugars, yeast, starches, fruit juices, refined grains, and processed meats. Sugar is the primary culprit and should be limited or avoided. See section 6.4 Anti-Yeast Diet for detailed references.

Attention

Section H: High Glutamate and Need for GABA and Vitamin B₆

Glutamate is a transmitter with excitatory effects in the brain. Excitatory glutamate converts to the calming neurotransmitter GABA. The amount of glutamate can increase in the brain if there is inefficiency in the glutamate decarboxylase enzyme or deficiency of vitamin B_6, which is necessary for the enzyme to function.

High glutamate is found in additives (MSG and aspartame are the most problematic) and in processed foods, milk products, grains, peanuts, and meats.

Poor attention can occur when glutamate is excessive and GABA is low. Other symptoms may include anxiety, irritability and sleep problems. The negative effects of glutamate in the brain are modulated by the calming amino acid and inhibitory neurotransmitter, GABA.

What to Do and How to Do It
- GABA absorbs best on an empty stomach, but may be taken with food.
- GABA's beneficial effects may affect dosing of medications used for ADHD, anxiety, and seizures. Do not add GABA without discussing it first with your child's prescribing physician.
- GABA should not be used if the child is already taking a medication that increases or potentially affects GABA, such as benzodiazepines, barbiturates, narcotics, and gabapentin.
- GABA, especially at higher doses, should only be used under the guidance of a health care practitioner.
- Side effects can include lethargy, excitability, and irritability.

GABA TOTAL DAILY GOAL DOSING

AGE	DOSE	FREQUENCY	TOTAL DAILY DOSE FROM ALL SOURCES
2 to 5	25 to 50 mg	2 times per day (breakfast and dinner)	50 to 100 mg
6 to 10	50 to 100 mg	2 times per day (breakfast and dinner)	100 to 200 mg
11 +	250 mg	1 or 2 times per day (breakfast and dinner)	250 to 500 mg

Vitamin B_6
Vitamin B_6 (pyridoxine) and its active form, pyridoxal-5'-phosphate (P5P), are necessary for the enzyme glutamate decarboxylase to convert excitatory glutamate to calming GABA. See section 4.5 The Worker B's, for B_6 dosing.

Section I: Histamine Reduction

Histamine is a chemical released by the body in allergic reactions and is usually associated with a runny nose, nasal congestion, postnasal drip, itchy eyes or nose, and skin rashes. Histamine is also an excitatory neurotransmitter that, when elevated, can increase inattention. Individuals who already have elevated neuronal histamine are more sensitive to the behavioral and attention-related effects of histamine-releasing reactions. Histamine may be a contributing factor if your child's symptoms suggest an allergy or if behavior worsens during the allergy season.

What to Do and How to Do It
Provided here is a brief summary on histamine. For thorough information and specific guidelines on dosing and side effects, see section 2.1 Allergies. Basic strategies include:

1. Removing the triggers for allergies
   - Inhalants (e.g., grass, trees, pollen, mold, animal danders)
   - Food that causes type I IgE histamine-releasing allergies
2. Using antihistamine medications
3. Taking supplements that reduce histamine release

SUPPLEMENTS THAT REDUCE HISTAMINE RELEASE

SUPPLEMENT	DESCRIPTION	AGE	DAILY DOSE	TOTAL DAILY DOSE FROM ALL SOURCES
Quercetin	Plant flavonol Anti-inflammatory	2 to 5	250 mg 2 times per day	500 mg
		6 to 10	500 mg 2 times per day	1,000 mg
		11 +	500 mg 2 times per day	1,000 mg
Pantothenic acid (vitamin B₅)	Water soluble B vitamin Nontoxic	2 to 5	100 to 250 mg per day	250 mg
		6 to 10	250 mg 2 or 3 times per day	750 mg
		11 +	500 mg 2 times per day	1,000 mg
Vitamin C (ascorbic acid)	Water soluble Nontoxic Excess causes loose stools	2 to 5	100 to 250 mg per day	250 mg
		6 to 10	250 mg 2 or 3 times per day	750 mg
		11 +	500 mg 2 times per day	1,000 mg

- Lower doses can be used for maintenance and reducing allergy potential.
- All three of the supplements may be taken together.
- Antihistamine supplements should not be taken when being skin tested for allergies.

■ *2.5 Communication and Language Delays*

Language and communication issues are part of the diagnostic criteria for autism. Language issues can sometimes be a coexisting issue for children with ADHD, who may have associated learning disabilities.

Communication

Symptoms/signs your child may exhibit
- Delayed or absent language
- Atypical language such as delayed echolalia (e.g. "scripting"—reciting, often verbatim—from movies, videos, songs, etc.)
- Difficulty with conversations
- Dyspraxia or apraxia (difficulty moving mouth, jaw, tongue, and lips automatically to produce intelligible speech)

Main possible nutritional contributing factors
- Food intolerances and opiate-like peptides
- Omega-3 deficiency
- Excess glutamate and need for GABA
- Hypomethylation, need for B_{12}, folinic acid, trimethylglycine/dimethylglycine
- Need for serotonin support
- Vitamin D deficiency
- Need for biotin

DETERMINING WHICH SUPPLEMENTS AND DIET CHANGES MAY BE HELPFUL

IF YOUR CHILD HAS LANGUAGE DELAYS AND SOME OF THE FOLLOWING SYMPTOMS	SEE THE APPLICABLE SECTION BELOW	DIETARY AND OTHER RECOMMENDATIONS	OTHER SOURCES FOR INFORMATION
Food cravings for milk casein and/or gluten and/or soy In a "fog" or "own world" Bowel problems Unexplained laughing High pain tolerance Poor eye contact Attention problems Mood problems	Section A: Food Intolerances and Elimination of Opioid Food Culprits	Section A: Food Intolerances and Elimination of Opioid Food Culprits Gluten-Free Casein-Free Soy-Free (GFCFSF) diet	Chapter 4: section 4.17 Digestive Enzymes Chapter 6: section 6.1 GFCFSF diet www.gfcfdiet.com
Cracking, peeling, chipping nails Attention problems Cognitive problems Vision dysfunction Skin: eczema, dermatitis Excessive thirst Hard earwax	Section B: Essential Omega-3 Fatty Acids		Chapter 4: section 4.15 Essential Omega-3 Fatty Acids
Tics Hyperactivity	Section C: High Glutamate and Need for GABA and Vitamin B_6	Limit/avoid glutamate (excitotoxins)	Chapter 4: section 4.11 GABA and Theanine and section 4.5 Vitamin B_6
Repetitive behaviors Perseverations Scripting OCD	Section D: Methylation Support		Chapter 2: section 2.3 Anxiety
Anxiety or OCD symptoms Depressed mood Sleep disruption Perseverations	Section E: Serotonin Support		Chapter 2: section 2.3 Anxiety

Scaly, cracked "ring around the mouth" Profuse sweating Delayed tooth eruption Bowing legs Bulging forehead "Knobby" knees or ankles	Section F: Vitamin D	Sun exposure, if tolerated	Chapter 4: section 4.2 Vitamin D
Picky appetite White lines on nails Frequent illness Eczema/dermatitis Developmental delays Growth delays Sensory sensitivities Inattention Highly refined "white" diet	Section G: Zinc	Good protein intake Low intake of refined carbohydrates	Chapter 4: section 4.9 Zinc

Communication

Section A: Food Intolerances and Elimination of Opioid Food Culprits

Food intolerances can cause communication and language delays. A full discussion of food intolerances is beyond the scope of this book. More information and resources are available in section 4.17 Digestive Enzymes and section 6.1 Gluten-Free Casein-Free Soy-Free (GFCFSF) Diet.

In short, food proteins, particularly those from milk (casein) and wheat (gluten), may be incompletely digested to peptides and may enter the bloodstream from the intestine via an abnormally permeable intestinal lining (referred to as "leaky gut"). These partially digested protein peptides can potentially cross the blood–brain barrier, negatively affecting brain function, including contributing to mood, attention, and behavior by several mechanisms:

- Blocking neurotransmitter messages
- Creating opiate-like doping effects from gluten (gliadorphin), milk casein (casomorphin), and soy
- Triggering brain inflammation

The most obvious symptom is craving for the food opiate sources (gluten, milk products, and soy). The opioid effect can contribute to language and communication delays and also inattention, poor eye contact, irritability, and increased self-stimulating behavior.

What to Do and How to Do It

Provided here is a brief summary of two main treatment strategies for food intolerances and the opioid effect.

1. GFCFSF Diet—Elimination Trial: the "gold standard" for treatment
   - The most common problem food proteins are gluten, milk casein, and soy.
   - Your child's body is the best test. Eliminate the food(s) to see whether behavior improves and reintroduce or challenge the body to see whether behavior worsens.

2. Digestive enzymes, including dipeptidyl peptidase-IV (DPP-IV)
   - More efficiently digest gluten; casein, soy, and other food proteins; carbohydrates; and fats.
   - Reduce the opioid load due to insufficient DPP-IV enzyme function; this can also "mimic" the diet.

Digestive Enzyme Supplements
See section 4.17 Digestive Enzymes for detailed information on specific enzyme products and dosing.

Section B: Essential Omega-3 Fatty Acids

The essential omega-3 fatty acids are EPA and DHA. Almost 60 percent of the brain is composed of fat, with DHA being the primary structural component of the human brain and retina. DHA also affects focus and attention.

What to Do and How to Do It
Provided here is a brief summary on omega-3 fatty acids. For thorough information and specific guidelines on supplement brands, dosing, and side effects, see section 4.15 Essential Omega-3 Fatty Acids.

The best food sources of omega-3 fatty acids are found in seafood. Those highest in mercury, PCBs, and other toxins include tomalley (crab mustard), farmed fish, trout, imported shrimp, and the large "steak" fish such as tuna, bluefish, swordfish, and shark. The safest choices include anchovies, sardines, domestic shrimp, rockfish, and tilapia. See the Environmental Working Group website, www.ewg.org, and the Environmental Defense Fund website, www.edf.org.

Omega-3 supplements
- For communication, language, and also focus and attention issues, we recommend that DHA amount be equal to or greater than the EPA.
- Use only direct-source EPA and DHA, which is more efficient than flaxseed-source ALA.
- Use toxin-free supplements: pharmaceutical grade or molecular distillation to remove toxins.

Types of high DHA supplements available in capsules, liquids, and chewables
- Cod liver oil (contains varying amounts of vitamins A and D)
- Fish oils with increased DHA to EPA ratio
- Vegetarian algae-source DHA

The following supplements have substantial levels of DHA:
- Barleans Omega Swirl
- Omega Cure (unflavored)
- Nordic Naturals ProOmega or Ultimate Omega
- Carlson Norwegian Cod Liver Oil with A and D_3
- Genestra Super DHA Liquid
- Nordic Naturals Baby's DHA (and EPA)
- Neuromins DHA caps (algae-source DHA)
- Nordic Naturals ProDHA 1,000 soft gels

OMEGA-3 EPA AND DHA TOTAL DAILY GOAL DOSING

AGE	EPA	DHA	FREQUENCY
2 to 5	200 to 400 mg	200 to 400 mg	Daily with food
6 to 10	500 to 650 mg	400 to 500 mg	Daily with food
11 +	500 to 800 mg	500 to 650 mg	Daily with food

- Though DHA is preferred for assisting in communication, attention, focus, eye contact, and mood, EPA is also important and should be included.
- Higher than recommended doses of omega-3 fatty acids should only be given under the guidance of a skilled health care practitioner.

Section C: High Glutamate and Need for GABA and Vitamin B₆

Glutamate is a transmitter with excitatory effects in the brain. Excitatory glutamate converts to the calming neurotransmitter GABA. The amount of glutamate can increase in the brain if there is inefficiency in the glutamate decarboxylase enzyme or deficiency of vitamin B_6, which is necessary for the enzyme to function.

High glutamate is found in additives (MSG and aspartame are the most problematic) and also in processed foods, milk products, grains, peanuts, and meats.

Poor attention can occur when glutamate is excessive and GABA is low. Other symptoms may include anxiety, irritability, and sleep problems. The negative effects of glutamate in the brain are modulated by the calming amino acid and inhibitory neurotransmitter, GABA.

What to Do and How to Do It
- GABA is best absorbed on an empty stomach, but can be taken with food.
- GABA's beneficial effects may affect dosing of medications used for ADHD, anxiety, and seizures. Do not add GABA without discussing it first with your child's prescribing physician.
- GABA should not be used if the child is already taking a medication that increases or potentially affects GABA, such as benzodiazepines, barbiturates, narcotics, and gabapentin.
- GABA, especially at higher doses, should only be used under the guidance of a health care practitioner.
- Side effects can include lethargy, excitability, and irritability.

GABA TOTAL DAILY GOAL DOSING

AGE	DOSE	FREQUENCY	TOTAL DAILY DOSE FROM ALL SOURCES
2 to 5	25 to 50 mg	2 times per day (breakfast and dinner)	50 to 100 mg
6 to 10	50 to 100 mg	2 times per day (breakfast and dinner)	100 to 200 mg
11 +	250 mg	1 or 2 times per day (breakfast and dinner)	250 to 500 mg

Communication

Vitamin B$_6$

Vitamin B$_6$ (pyridoxine) and its active form, pyridoxal-5'-phosphate (P5P), are necessary for the enzyme glutamate decarboxylase to convert excitatory glutamate to calming GABA.

What to Do and How to Do It

Some multiple vitamin supplements will have B$_6$ and/or P5P, which may be sufficient and not require additional supplementation. If they are not being used, supplementation may be necessary. See Section D: Methylation Support for dosing.

Section D: Methylation Support

Methylation is a biochemical process critical in gene expression, DNA synthesis, synchronizing neuron firing, toxic metal metabolism, regulation of protein function and RNA metabolism, and creation of cellular energy. Methylation deficit is called undermethylation or hypomethylation. Excess methylation is called overmethylation or hypermethylation.

The methylation pathway is involved in the metabolism of methionine and homocysteine and requires the donation of chemicals called methyl groups. Details of this pathway are discussed in section 3.2 Mechanisms: Methylation.

According to William J. Walsh, Ph.D., of the Walsh Research Institute, hypomethylation occurs in more than 95 percent of people with autism, more than 99 percent in people with ADHD with an oppositional defiant presentation, and 20 to 30 percent of other ADHD presentations.

In autism (and to a lesser degree in ADHD), it is not uncommon to find a gene mutation—MTHFR (methylenetetrahydrofolate reductase)—that renders the individual dependent on therapeutic doses of the methylation nutrients.

What to Do and How to Do It

Provided here is a brief summary on the nutrients important in methylation: B$_6$, B$_{12}$, folinic acid, DMG, and TMG For thorough information and specific guidelines on dosing and side effects, see section 4.5 Methylation Nutrients.

Problems in the methylation pathway and possible need for dimethylglycine (DMG) or trimethylglycine (TMG) are more prevalent in children with autism and are seen in a subset of children with ADHD.

Testing for B$_6$, B$_{12}$, and folinic acid deficiency should be accomplished by a skilled health care practitioner. Serum levels of these vitamins are not sensitive markers for deficiency and do not decline until extreme late stages of deficiency. There are specialized metabolite tests that are more specific for functional status.

Use B vitamins for methylation support. Multiple vitamin and B complex supplements may or may not have sufficient levels of these B vitamins. Added doses may be required.

Vitamin B$_6$

- P5P is the active cofactor form
- B$_6$ is more effective if taken with magnesium
- If sulfation is defective as is the case with phenol sensitivities/intolerances, avoid the P5P form of B$_6$.
- Absorption can be hindered by antacids.
- Higher doses require the guidance of a health care practitioner.

VITAMIN B$_6$ AND P5P TOTAL DAILY GOAL DOSING

FORM OF B$_6$	AGE	DAILY DOSE WITH FOOD BEFORE NOON	TOTAL DAILY DOSE FROM ALL SOURCES
Vitamin B$_6$ (pyridoxine)	2 to 5	10 to 15 mg	30 mg
	6 to 10	20 to 30 mg	60 mg
	11 +	50 mg	100 mg
P5P (Pyridoxal-5′-phosphate)	2 to 5	5 mg	5 mg
	6 to 10	10 mg	10 mg
	11 +	15 mg	15 mg

Vitamin B$_{12}$

- Methylcobalamin and hydroxocobalamin are active forms that have excellent bioavailability.
- Poor absorption and/or the use of antacids can cause B$_{12}$ deficiency.
- Sublingual forms may be preferred (they bypass the stomach and small intestine).
- Higher doses require the guidance of a health care practitioner.

METHYL B$_{12}$ TOTAL DAILY GOAL DOSING

AGE	DAILY DOSE WITH FOOD BEFORE NOON	TOTAL DAILY DOSE FROM ALL SOURCES
2 to 5	50 to 100 mcg	100 mcg
6 to 10	100 to 500 mcg	500 mcg
11 +	500 to 1000 mcg	1,000 mcg

Folinic acid

- Folinic acid is one of the preferred folate forms that is noted for its excellent bioavailability.
- Folic acid is least effective and best avoided.
- Absorption can be hindered by antacids, antiseizure medications, and tetracycline.
- Folinic acid can mask the symptoms of pernicious anemia due to B$_{12}$ deficiency. This can be avoided through appropriate testing and pairing folinic acid with vitamin B$_{12}$ supplementation.
- Higher doses require the guidance of a health care practitioner.

Communication

FOLINIC ACID TOTAL DAILY GOAL DOSING

AGE	DAILY DOSE WITH OR WITHOUT FOOD	TOTAL DAILY DOSE FROM ALL SOURCES
2 to 5	100 mcg	100 mcg
6 to 10	200 mcg	200 mcg
11 +	400 mcg	400 mcg

DMG and TMG
- Both have methyl groups attached to the amino acid glycine.
- Both provide methyl groups.
- Both have been demonstrated to improve language, cognition, and eye contact, and reduce echolalia, anxiety, and obsessive–compulsive behaviors.
- Not all individuals tolerate DMG and/or TMG.

DMG has two methyl groups:
- It is ideal to include folinic acid first.
- If folate function is insufficient, DMG may cause increased irritability, self-stimulating behavior, or hyperactivity.
- DMG can have a positive effect on speech, eye contact, and cognition.
- Higher doses require the guidance of a health care practitioner.

DMG TOTAL DAILY GOAL DOSING

AGE	DOSE	FREQUENCY	TOTAL DAILY DOSE FROM ALL SOURCES
2 to 5	125 mg	1 time per day	125 mg
6 to 10	125 mg	2 times per day	250 mg
11 +	250 mg	2 times per day	500 mg

TMG has three methyl groups
- When TMG donates a methyl group, it becomes DMG.
- TMG can have positive results on speech and eye contact.
- If TMG results in side effects, adding taurine may improve tolerance.
- Higher doses require the guidance of a health care practitioner.

TMG TOTAL DAILY GOAL DOSING

AGE	DOSE	FREQUENCY	TOTAL DAILY DOSE FROM ALL SOURCES
2 to 5	175 mg	2 times per day	350 mg
6 to 10	250 mg	2 times per day	500 mg
11 +	500 mg	2 times per day	1,000 mg

What Else Should I Know?
All supplements come in liquid, capsule, and tablet forms. Refer to section 4.5 Methylation Nutrients.

- Side effects of any of the methylation nutrients can include increased activity, stimming, irritability, or anxiety. These are more likely to occur in children who are overmethylated. If these symptoms occur, stop the supplement and discuss with your health care practitioner.
- Side effects of TMG can occur in children who do not have enough taurine and may respond well when it is added. If your child has side effects, adding taurine may be helpful. See section 4.12 Taurine for dosing.
- If your child has an autism disorder, only use taurine under the guidance of a health care practitioner. A subset of children with autism and a smaller subset with ADHD have metabolic disorders, some of which may render them intolerant to specific amino acids, including taurine.

Section E: Serotonin Support

Serotonin is an important transmitter in the brain that affects communication, language and also cognition, attention, mood, and behavior. The amino acid tryptophan converts to 5-hydroxytryptophan (5-HTP), which then converts to serotonin; serotonin then converts further to melatonin (the hormone that affects sleep).

The following are the primary nutrients critical in these pathways: magnesium, zinc, iron, methylation support (B_6, B_{12}, folinic acid), and tryptophan-sparing vitamin B_3 (niacinamide). Low levels of serotonin can result in delays in language and social skills, particularly in children with autism. It can also result in anxiety, obsessive–compulsive symptoms, depression, self-stimulatory behaviors, repetitive movements, and sleep disorders.

What to Do and How to Do It

There are three main ways to raise serotonin:

1. Medications such as Selective Serotonin Reuptake Inhibitors (SSRIs)
   - SSRIs and 5-HTP raise serotonin levels in the brain but by different mechanisms.
   - Serotonin is released by neurons (nerve cells) in the brain and taken back up by these cells in order to be reused.
   - SSRIs block this uptake so that the serotonin effect is prolonged.
   - SSRIs must be prescribed and monitored by a physician.
2. Direct nutritional support of the serotonin pathway via L-tryptophan and 5-HTP
   - 5-HTP supplementation produces more serotonin directly as compared to L-tryptophan.
   - Use 5-HTP under the care of a knowledgeable health care practitioner.
   - The use of only tryptophan and/or 5-HTP is not recommended when taking an SSRI medication because there is the risk for excessive serotonin.
   - Opposite reactions such as hyperactivity or insomnia, and/or manic symptoms may occur.

Communication

3. Serotonin nutrient cofactor supplementation:
   - Magnesium, zinc, iron, methylation support (B_6, B_{12}, and folinic acid), and vitamin B_3

These nutrients are essential to optimal serotonin metabolism. Use of a good multivitamin is a start for providing these nutrient cofactors. More specific adjustment of nutrients is best done with guidance by a skilled health care practitioner (physician or nutritionist).

Section F: Vitamin D

Vitamin D deficiency can result in developmental delays including communication and language delay. Vitamin D is also important in skin health, immunity, bone health, and hormone regulation. Risk factors for the development of vitamin D deficiency include inadequate sun exposure (or use of sunblock), darker skin pigmentation, obesity, breast feeding, low dietary intake, and fat malabsorption.

What to Do and How to Do It
Provided here is a brief summary on vitamin D. See chapter 4 for more information on functions, products, dosing, and side effects.

Vitamin D supplements
- Vitamin D_3 is available in capsules, tablets, and liquids.
- The micellized version of vitamin D_3 is a water-soluble form of vitamin D that is well absorbed and especially useful in conditions where absorption is poor.
- Vitamin D_3 (cholecalciferol) is the best form to use for supplementation.
- Vitamin D_2 (ergocalciferol) converts to vitamin D_3 and is less effective long term.
- The oil and micellized forms are preferred over the dry forms.

VITAMIN D TOTAL DAILY GOAL DOSING

AGE	TOTAL DAILY DOSE FROM ALL SOURCES
2 to 5	400 to 600 IU
6 to 10	600 to 800 IU
11 +	800 to 2,000 IU

- The total daily dose includes all sources such as from cod liver oil and multiple vitamins.
- Have blood testing (25-hydroxy vitamin D) to guide dosing. The optimal goal level is 60 to 80 ng/mL.
- Adequate vitamin A intake must be maintained. See section 4.1 Vitamin A for dosing.
- Higher doses may be required due to poor absorption or lab findings. This should be accomplished with a skilled health care practitioner.

Section G: Zinc

Zinc deficiency can result in communication and language delays as well as poor eye contact, sensory deficits, picky appetite, skin conditions, and poor glucose control.

Zinc deficiency can stem from poor intake, higher needs, and/or depletion by a glycemic diet, medications, or toxins.

What to Do and How to Do It

Provided here is a brief summary on zinc. For thorough information and specific guidelines on dosing and side effects, see section 4.9 Zinc.

Zinc supplements
- Well tolerated: gluconates, chelates, citrates, acetates, picolinates, chlorides, and bisglycinates
- Strong taste, needs disguising: sulfates

ZINC TOTAL DAILY GOAL DOSING

AGE	DOSE	FREQUENCY	TOTAL DAILY DOSE FROM ALL SOURCES
2 to 5	5 to 10 mg	1 or 2 times per day	10 to 20 mg
6 to 10	10 mg	2 times per day	20 mg
11 +	10 to 15 mg	2 times per day	20 to 30 mg

For optimal oral absorption, an empty stomach is best, but it may not be feasible if nausea occurs. Large doses can cause gastric discomfort, nausea, and inhibit the digestive enzyme DPP-IV (which digests opioids from gluten and casein). In addition:
- Avoid or limit giving oral zinc at the same time as interfering nutrients such as calcium, iron, folate, and phosphorylated nutrients (R5P, P5P, phosphatidylcholine); this may not always be feasible.
- Consider topical zinc lotion such as Kirkman Labs (22 mg of zinc per scoop). Apply to muscle areas in which absorption is highest: shoulders, back, or the calves.
- Zinc excess can lower copper levels. Copper levels need to be maintained.
- Use the Zinc Tally Taste Test in section 4.9 for evaluating progress with zinc supplementation.
- Higher doses may be required because of poor absorption, antacid use, the presence of toxic metals in the body, or lab findings. This should be accomplished with a skilled health care practitioner.

■ *2.6 Constipation*

Constipation is common in children with autism. It may also be seen in some children with ADHD and other behavioral or developmental disorders. Constipation can contribute to both physical discomfort and behavioral symptoms.

Constipation

Symptoms/signs your child may exhibit

- Infrequent stools (stools should occur daily)
- Hard, difficult-to-pass stools
- Small, pellet-like stools
- Abdominal discomfort, bloating, and/or distension
- Posturing (applying pressure to the lower abdomen)

Main possible contributing nutritional factors

- Poor hydration
- Low fiber
- Magnesium deficiency
- Vitamin C deficiency
- Insufficient or poor quality bile
- Elevated opiate-like peptides from casein or gluten
- Delayed motility

DETERMINING WHICH SUPPLEMENTS AND DIET CHANGES MAY BE HELPFUL

IF YOUR CHILD HAS CONSTIPATION AND ONE OR MORE OF THE FOLLOWING SYMPTOMS	SEE THE APPLICABLE SECTION BELOW	DIETARY AND OTHER RECOMMENDATIONS	OTHER SOURCES FOR INFORMATION
Hard, dry stool Inadequate fluid intake Dry/chapped lips Dark/concentrated urine Dizziness or lightheadedness	Section A: Hydration	Section A: Hydration	
Hard, dry stools	Section B: Fiber	Section B: Fiber	
Delayed intestinal motility Hyperactivity Repetitive behaviors Sound sensitivity Anxiety	Section C: Magnesium		Chapter 4: section 4.8 Magnesium and Calcium
Frequent colds or illnesses	Section D: Vitamin C		Chapter 4: section 4.7 Vitamin C
Yellow or gritty/sandy stools Anxiety Tics Seizures	Section E: Taurine		Chapter 4: section 4.12 Taurine
Food cravings for milk casein and/or gluten and/or soy In a "fog" or "own world" Unexplained laughing High pain tolerance Poor eye contact Mood problems Attention problems Language delays	Section F: Food Intolerances and Elimination of Opioid Food Culprits	Section F: Food Intolerances and Elimination of Opioid Food Culprits Gluten-Free Casein-Free Soy-Free (GFCFSF) diet	Chapter 4: section 4.17 Digestive Enzymes Chapter 6: section 6.1 GFCFSF Diet

Constipation can have wide-ranging effects on both physical and behavioral functioning. Constipation can understandably contribute to stomach aches and general discomfort. The pressure on the stomach from excessive stools in the large intestine can worsen reflux symptoms and contribute to urinary frequency or urine accidents. If constipation is significant enough, it can also lead to decreased appetite.

From a functional medicine perspective, bowel movement function is the elimination of toxins. Toxins are generated daily from the body's normal metabolic processes and need to be eliminated either through breath, sweat, urine, or stool. If stools do not occur daily, toxins are not eliminated and can be reabsorbed. This overburdens the body with "old" toxins, reducing the ability to remove the new toxins generated and leading to an increased total body load of toxins. This can lead to behavioral symptoms that may be improved by regular stool elimination. As our pharmacist colleague Lyn Shumake is fond of saying, "You should think of your intestine as short-term parking, not long-term parking; no one stays overnight in the garage."

The treatment goal outlined in this section is at least one daily bowel movement that is formed, even in color, easily passed, and free of undigested food and mucous.

Section A: Hydration

A common contributing factor to constipation is poor hydration. Most people, not just children with ADHD or autism, do not drink adequate amounts of fluids. There are a number of both physical and behavioral symptoms of dehydration, including the symptoms described in the chart on page 72. It is important to provide adequate hydration so the following nutritional supplement recommendations can be helpful. For example, magnesium and vitamin C work in part by pulling fluid into the large intestine. It is difficult to hydrate the stools adequately if the body itself is not well hydrated.

In addition to not taking in sufficient fluids, there are foods or drinks that may themselves be dehydrating. Caffeinated drinks such as sodas, coffee, or teas all have diuretic effects and are dehydrating, as are very sugary drinks.

What to Do and How to Do It
Water is the absolute best fluid to use for hydration. If your child refuses water, try giving water flavored with as little amount of juice as possible. About 70 to 80 percent of total fluid intake comes from drinking water and other non-soda beverages. The rest is obtained from foods, especially vegetables and fruits.

The common sports electrolyte drinks have negligible electrolytes. They also contain artificial coloring and additives that have been noted to increase hyperactive behavior in children. The usual pediatric electrolyte solutions contain electrolytes but also have artificial sweeteners (such as Sucralose), flavoring, and coloring.

The ideal natural electrolyte solution is coconut water, a sterile solution inside the coconut. It is a 100 percent natural vitamin and mineral electrolyte solution. It is the perfect natural electrolyte drink served plain or with some added natural juice to flavor. It is available commercially as a refreshing drink.

How Much Fluid Should My Child Drink?
Fluid intake includes water, vegetable juices, electrolyte drinks (coconut water), herb teas, and fruit juices (not sodas). These recommendations are for daily "added fluid," which is in addition to a diet that includes high-moisture foods (melons, tomatoes, fruits, lettuces, and soups).

DAILY FLUID CONSUMPTION RECOMMENDATIONS

AGE	DAILY AMOUNT	AMOUNT IN OUNCES
2 to 5	4 to 5 cups	32 to 40
6 to 10	5 to 7 cups	40 to 56
11 +	7 to 11 cups	56 to 88

What Else Should I Know?
It is better to add water or electrolyte solutions in small amounts frequently. Allow thirst to be satisfied and avoid forcing excess water consumption. In infants, be careful not to overhydrate with water, as this can lead to a serious condition called hyponatremia, in which the body's sodium levels are too low.

Urinating fewer than three times per day can be a sign of inadequate hydration or dehydration. Observing urine color can also be helpful. If the urine is dark yellow or brown, then it is possible there is dehydration. This is not to be confused with the bright yellow urine color that can occur when taking supplements, especially B vitamins.

Section B: Fiber

Dietary fiber is essential to healthy digestive function and to the milieu (living organisms) that are critical to digestive and systemic health. Fiber is present in plant foods only.

What to Do and How to Do It
There are two types of fiber:

Insoluble fiber, which will not dissolve in liquids. Sources include whole grains, nuts, seeds, beans, vegetables, and the edible skins of fruits and vegetables. This type of fiber draws water into the stool and has a bulking and cleansing action. It is not physiologically active.

Soluble fiber, which is completely soluble in liquids. Sources include legumes, oat bran (gluten-free), nuts, seeds, fruits, and guar gum. Soluble fiber absorbs water, which improves stool quality and is helpful in treating constipation and diarrhea. It provides prebiotic "fuel" for beneficial colonic fermentation by good flora, leading to important physiologically active byproducts including nutrient manufacture (biotin and vitamin K).

It is best to increase the foods that have fiber. However, this can be difficult in those whose appetites are limited. We offer two suggestions:

1. Add (hide) vegetable and fruit purees in meatballs, pancakes, muffins, spaghetti sauce, and fruit smoothies. This is the "Trojan Horse Technique"

described in our book *The Kid-Friendly ADHD & Autism Cookbook*. See also Section 2.13 Picky Eating.

2. Add gluten-free casein-free soy-free (GFCFSF) soluble fiber such as guar gum, which dissolves like sugar in liquids and has no distinguishable taste or texture as compared to the gelatinous psyllium fiber. Soluble fiber mixes well in water, vegetable juice, and smoothies. It improves stool consistency and is helpful in resolving constipation and diarrhea.

FIBER TOTAL DAILY GOAL DOSING

AGE	DAILY AMOUNT
2 to 5	19 to 20 grams
6 to 10	20 to 25 grams
11 +	25 to 30 grams

Guar gum (pure, GFCFSF) can be added as part of the total daily fiber intake: 1 Tbs = 4 grams of fiber

GUAR GUM TOTAL DAILY GOAL DOSING

AGE	DAILY AMOUNT	TOTAL AMOUNT IN GRAMS OF FIBER
2 to 5	1 Tbs	4 grams
6 to 10	1 Tbs	4 grams
11 +	1 Tbs 2 times per day	8 grams

What Side Effects Should I Watch for?
If fiber is excessive, there can be increased flatulence (gas). If the smell of the gas and/or stool is extremely strong, it can indicate poor gut flora and a possible overgrowth of pathogens or an infection.

What Else Should I Know?
It is better to introduce the fiber slowly and observe the changes in bowel habits. Water consumption is essential. Inadequate water consumption when taking fiber supplements can cause constipation.

Fiber supplements, including guar gum, are best given one hour or more away from supplements or medications, as they can act as binders and inhibit the absorption of supplements and medications.

Section C: Magnesium
Magnesium can reduce or resolve constipation. It is calming and can reduce hyperactivity, stimming, perseverations, and anxiety. It is primarily found in green leafy vegetables. Intake of these vegetables is commonly insufficient in children with ADHD or autism spectrum disorders. The "picky appetite," which is more prevalent in children with autism than ADHD, leads to aversions for leafy greens and vegetables. Magnesium is also not easily absorbed, especially if there are digestive problems and/or the use of antacids.

According to Sidney MacDonald Baker, M.D., Ph.D., of all the remedies for constipation, magnesium citrate is the most effective. When there is magnesium deficiency, constipation is a common consequence. When the constipation is resolved via magnesium, then the underlying unmet need for magnesium has been corrected.

Magnesium improves stool function through two mechanisms:

1. It relaxes neuromuscular tension, allowing for the stools to move through more easily.
2. It pulls water into the large intestine and hydrates the stools; however, this occurs only after the body's "magnesium bank account" status has improved. The level called "bowel tolerance" is the amount that has a laxative effect and a gurgling rush of bowel sounds. When this occurs, reduce the dose to the amount that produces one to three easy-to-eliminate, soft, formed stools per day.

What to Do and How to Do It

Provided here is a brief summary on magnesium. For thorough information, products and specific guidelines, see section 4.8 Magnesium and Calcium.

Magnesium supplements
- Gentle (less laxative) stool effect: chelates, aspartates, glycinates, gluconates, and bisglycinates
- Laxative stool effect: citrates, chlorides, and sulfates

MAGNESIUM TOTAL DAILY GOAL DOSING

AGE	DOSE	FREQUENCY	TOTAL DAILY DOSE FROM ALL SOURCES
2 to 5	100 mg	1 or 2 times per day	200 mg
6 to 10	100 mg	2 or 3 times per day	300 mg
11 +	100 to 150 mg	2 or 3 times per day	450 mg

- Start at one-quarter to one-half of the recommended dose and increase the dose gradually every one to two days.
- The goal is the level that results in a healthy, easy-to-eliminate stool and avoids diarrhea.
- Diarrhea can cause a loss of magnesium.
- Watch for possible side effects and decrease the dose accordingly.
- If symptoms improve at lower than the goal dose, you may not need to continue to increase the dose.
- For higher than recommended doses, consult with a health care practitioner.

Calcium

Make sure calcium intake, either through diet or supplement, is adequate. Magnesium intake can lower calcium, and calcium intake can lower magnesium. It is important to have balance. If your child is not getting sufficient calcium from diet, a calcium supplement is indicated.

CALCIUM TOTAL DAILY GOAL DOSING

AGE	DOSE	FREQUENCY	TOTAL DAILY DOSE FROM ALL SOURCES
2 to 5	250 mg	2 times per day	500 mg
6 to 10	250 mg	3 times per day	750 mg
11 +	500 to 600 mg	2 times per day	1,000 to 1,200 mg

Section D: Vitamin C

Vitamin C (ascorbic acid) is a water-soluble antioxidant that is important in immunity, collagen, neurotransmitter function, and more. It also helps hydrate stools by pulling water into the large intestine.

What to Do and How to Do It
We would recommend looking for a supplement that only contains vitamin C. Some vitamin C products also contain other immune-supporting nutrients. It is best to use a pure vitamin C supplement as ascorbic acid to avoid potential overdosing of other nutrients that may be included. We recommend:
• Vitamin C 250 mg Hypoallergenic capsules, made by Kirkman Labs
• Pure ascorbic acid (pharmaceutical grade)

How Do I Dose Vitamin C?
Vitamin C can be taken regularly at maintenance doses, with increases based on need. The dose range is wide and has been found safe at doses as high as 10,000 mg or more.

Vitamin C is nontoxic because it is water soluble and self-limiting. When there is deficiency, higher need, stress, or illness, the absorption of vitamin C increases, resulting in less effect to the stool. As the need declines, less will be absorbed and the more likely there will be loose stools. For this reason, the dose required for constipation can vary in an individual, depending upon other current health conditions.

As described in the previous section on magnesium, vitamin C also pulls water into the large intestine and hydrates the stools; however, this occurs only after the body's needs are being met. As internal tissue status improves, less vitamin C is absorbed, allowing for the stool hydrating effect. The goal is to determine "bowel tolerance" and then reduce the dose to the amount that results in one or two formed soft stools daily—without diarrhea and the loud gurgling rush of bowel sounds.

VITAMIN C TOTAL DAILY GOAL DOSING

AGE	DOSE	FREQUENCY
2 to 5	250 to 500 mg	1 or 2 times per day
6 to 10	500 mg	1 or 2 times per day
11 +	1,000 mg	1 or 2 times per day

Constipation

- Start at half of the lowest recommended dose and increase as tolerated until the stool improves.
- The goal is "bowel tolerance"—the level that results in a healthy, easy-to-eliminate stool and avoids diarrhea.
- Watch for possible side effects and decrease the dose accordingly.
- If symptoms improve at lower than the goal dose, you may not need to continue to increase the dose.
- For higher than recommended doses, consult with a health care practitioner.

What Side Effects Should I Watch for?

The main limiting side effect of vitamin C is diarrhea or loose stools. Increase the dose gradually in order to determine your child's tolerance to vitamin C. Cut back on the dose and/or frequency when the stools are too loose.

What Else Should I Know?

Vitamin C is contraindicated in the following conditions. Please consult with a physician or specialist.

- Kidney disease of any kind
- Oxalate kidney stone formation (increases with vitamin C use)
- Hemochromatosis (iron storage disease)
- G6PD deficiency (inherited disorder affecting red blood cells)

Vitamin C supplements often contain corn. If your child has a food sensitivity to corn, you will need a corn-free version.

Section E: Taurine

Bile is produced in the liver as conjugated bile salts that are stored in the gallbladder. Prior to secretion, bile acids are combined (conjugated) with taurine or glycine and are released in the form of bile salts. One of the most common bile salts contains taurine (taurocholic acid). In response to fat intake, bile is released from the gallbladder into the small intestine to assist in fat digestion and absorption. Bile promotes intestinal motility; insufficient or ineffective bile can contribute to constipation. Bile also gives stools their normal brown color. When there is not enough bile, stools may be yellow or light tan. They may also appear sandy or gritty because bile salts have not bound to taurine.

What to Do and How to Do It

We recommend not using taurine without the guidance of a health care practitioner, especially if your child has an autism spectrum disorder. Some children with autism have metabolic disorders that result in problems in certain enzyme pathways or the ability to handle certain foods such as proteins. If there is a rare metabolic problem with the handling of proteins, giving additional amino acids such as taurine may be contraindicated. We usually recommend blood testing for amino acid levels as well as a metabolic workup (to the degree determined necessary by a health care practitioner) before using taurine.

TAURINE TOTAL DAILY GOAL DOSING

AGE	DOSE	FREQUENCY	TOTAL DAILY DOSE FROM ALL SOURCES
2 to 5	150 mg	1 or 2 times per day	300 mg
6 to 10	150 mg	2 times per day	300 mg
11 +	250 mg	2 times per day	500 mg

- Start at half of the lowest recommended dose and increase as tolerated until the stool improves.
- Watch for possible side effects and decrease the dose accordingly.
- If symptoms improve at lower than the goal dose, you may not need to continue to increase the dose.

What Side Effects Should I Watch for?
The main side effect of taurine can be diarrhea or loose stools. Increasing the dose gradually will help determine your child's level of tolerance.

What Else Should I Know?
Taurine improves magnesium function and has an overall calming effect on the nervous system. It may be helpful for lowering anxiety in some children. It also may be helpful for treatment of motor tics. Last, taurine is also reported to have antiseizure benefits.

Section F: Food Intolerances and Elimination of Opioid Food Culprits
Constipation can be a side effect of food intolerances. A full discussion of food intolerances is beyond the scope of this book. More information and resources are available in section 4.17 Digestive Enzymes and section 6.1 Gluten-Free Casein-Free Soy-Free (GFCFSF) Diet.

In short, food proteins, particularly those from milk (casein) and wheat (gluten), may be incompletely digested to peptides and may enter the bloodstream from the intestine via an abnormally permeable intestinal lining (referred to as "leaky gut"). These partially digested protein peptides can potentially cross the blood–brain barrier, negatively affecting brain function, including contributing to mood, attention, and behavior by several mechanisms:
- Blocking neurotransmitter messages
- Creating opiate-like doping effects from gluten (gliadorphin), milk casein (casomorphin), and soy
- Triggering brain inflammation

The most obvious symptom is a craving for the food opiate sources (gluten, milk products, and soy). In addition to constipation, other symptoms include inattention, poor focus, language delays, poor eye contact, irritability, and increased activity of repeated self-stimulatory behaviors. Effects may occur within an hour of consumption or be delayed up to seventy-two hours.

Constipation

What to Do and How to Do It

Provided here is a brief summary of two main treatment strategies for food intolerances and the opiate-like peptide effect.

1. Gluten-free Casein-free Soy-free (GFCFSF) Diet—Elimination Trial: the "gold standard" for treatment
   - The most common problem food proteins are gluten, milk casein, and soy.
   - Your child's body is the best test. Eliminate the food(s) to see whether behavior improves and reintroduce or challenge the body to see whether behavior worsens.
2. Digestive enzymes, including dipeptidyl peptidase-IV (DPP-IV)
   - More efficiently digest gluten, casein, soy, and other food proteins, carbohydrates, and fats.
   - Reduce the opioid load due to insufficient DPP-IV enzyme function; this can also "mimic" the diet.

Digestive Enzyme Supplements

See section 4.17 Digestive Enzymes for detailed information on specific enzyme products and dosing.

■ 2.7 Diarrhea

Children with autism frequently have GI issues, including diarrhea. Diarrhea can result in nutrient depletion. It can also be a sign of food intolerances, an underlying infectious condition that can occur from pathogens and/or parasites, or an inflammatory condition.

Symptoms/signs your child may exhibit
- Loose stools
- Frequent unformed stools
- Fatty stools
- Unusually foul-smelling stools

Main possible contributing factors
- Infections: bacterial, viral, or parasitic
- Intestinal imbalance of bacteria and/or yeast overgrowth
- Lactose and other disaccharide intolerances
- Food intolerances and opiate-like peptides (e.g., casein, gluten, soy)
- Fat malabsorption

DETERMINING WHICH SUPPLEMENTS AND DIET CHANGES MAY BE HELPFUL

IF YOUR CHILD HAS DIARRHEA AND SOME OF THE FOLLOWING SYMPTOMS	SEE THE APPLICABLE SECTION BELOW	DIETARY AND OTHER RECOMMENDATIONS	OTHER SOURCES OF INFORMATION
Fever Stool blood or mucous Poor fluid intake Poor growth Joint pains Abdominal pain Distention	Section A: Medical Causes		
Recurrent antibiotic use Oral thrush Yeast diaper rashes Skin conditions Poor hair quality Immune dysfunction	Section B: Treatment of Intestinal Yeast Overgrowth	Section B: Treatment of Intestinal Yeast Overgrowth Anti-yeast diet Fermented foods	Chapter 4: section 4.16 Probiotics and section 4.6 Biotin Chapter 6: section 6.4 Anti-Yeast Diet
Problems with cow's milk products, most sugars, and starches Gas/flatulence Bloating	Section C: Treatment of Lactose and Other Disaccharide Intolerances	Avoid disaccharide foods via the Specific Carbohydrate Diet (SCD) and Gut and Psychology Syndrome (GAPS) diets	Chapter 6: section 6.3 SCD and GAPS Diet
Food cravings for milk casein, and/or gluten, and/or soy In a "fog" or "own world" Unexplained laughing High pain tolerance Poor eye contact Mood problems Inattention Language delays	Section D: Food Intolerances and Elimination of Opioid Food Culprits	Section D: Food Intolerances and Elimination of Opioid Food Culprits Gluten-Free Casein-Free Soy-Free (GFCFSF) diet	Chapter 4: section 4.17 Digestive Enzymes Chapter 6: section 6.1 GFCFSF Diet
Stools that: Float Appear fatty, slick, foamy Have a rancid foul smell Are tan, yellow, or gray	Section E: Treatment of Fat Malabsorption	Section E: Treatment of Fat Malabsorption	Chapter 4: section 4.17 Digestive Enzymes *Digestive Wellness*, 4th ed., by Elizabeth Lipski

Diarrhea

Section A: Medical Causes

We strongly recommend a thorough evaluation by your child's primary care provider to rule out medical causes. These can include common viral or parasitic infections, bacterial infections, overflow loose stools because of unsuspected constipation, celiac disease, and inflammatory bowel conditions such as colitis. The supplement and diet recommendations do not replace medical care. Inform the physician about any diet and supplement changes and the effects of those changes.

Your physician may request testing or may treat the most common causes of chronic diarrhea such as food reactions, increased bowel motility, and imbalanced bowel flora (inadequate good flora and/or excessive yeast or pathogen overgrowth). If your child does not respond to medical treatment, diet changes, and/or probiotics, let your child's physician know so he or she can determine whether further workup or referral to a specialist is indicated.

In a subset of children with autism, inflammatory bowel disease is present. If you have a child with autism whose diarrhea does not have an identifiable cause and whose symptoms do not respond to treatments, consider consulting a GI specialist familiar with the digestive problems unique to autism.

Section B: Treatment of Intestinal Yeast Overgrowth

Imbalanced bacteria in the intestine can allow overgrowth of yeast or pathogenic (disease-causing) bacteria in the intestine. This can result in diarrhea.

What to Do and How to Do It

Provided here is a summary on probiotics and treatments for yeast overgrowth. For more thorough information, see section 2.18 Yeast Overgrowth, section 4.16 Probiotics, and section 6.4 Anti-Yeast Diet.

Main beneficial treatments
- Probiotics (beneficial bacteria)
- Biotin
- Antifungal (anti-yeast) medications or herbs
- Anti-yeast diet

Probiotics

Probiotics are beneficial live microorganisms called the microbiome, found throughout the body including in the intestinal tract. There are more than 100 trillion good bacteria in the body with 500 to 1,000 different species (forty to fifty of which are main species) in the human gut. These beneficial bacteria maintain healthy flora, prevent overgrowth of harmful pathogens and yeast, and also produce healthy nutrients. For a complete listing of probiotic benefits, specific products, and dosing guideliens, see section 4.16 Probiotics.

Biotin

Biotin is a water-soluble B vitamin, manufactured in the human digestive tract by healthy flora. Antibiotics depress biotin production, which leads to yeast/fungal overgrowth and diarrhea. Biotin helps keep yeast in a less invasive form, which makes yeast easier to eradicate. Biotin is one of the safest supplements. It has no toxicity at any level. See section 4.6 The Helper B: Biotin, for more information and dosing guidelines.

Antifungal Medications or Herbs

Probiotics help provide beneficial bacteria to the intestinal tract but do not directly kill yeast. To bring yeast levels back down to normal levels, antifungal medications and/or herbs are used. Probiotics then help maintain good bacterial balance to help prevent yeast overgrowth from recurring.

Antifungal treatments may include herbs and/or prescription medications. Depending on the amount of yeast present, intestinal symptoms and behavioral side effects from treatment may be significant. Known as "yeast die-off" symptoms, these may include irritability, behavioral regression, and flu-like symptoms. Because of the potential for significant side effects, antifungal treatment should be guided by a health care practitioner based on your child's history and, where possible, specific testing for yeast. See section 2.18 Yeast Overgrowth.

Anti-Yeast Diet
The anti-yeast diet prohibits foods that feed yeast: sugars, yeast, starches, fruit juices, refined grains, and processed meats. Sugar is the primary culprit to limit or avoid. See section 6.4 Anti-Yeast Diet for detailed references.

Section C: Treatment of Lactose and Other Disaccharide Intolerances

Many children with autism and some children with ADHD have damage to the GI tract, which causes poor production of digestive enzymes, including enzymes that break down sugars. Disaccharidase enzymes digest disaccharide "double sugars" into simple monosaccharide "single sugars." Monosaccharide single sugars are easy to digest and do not require enzymes. The failure to break down the double sugars results in gas, bloating, yeast overgrowth, and diarrhea. The greater the damage to the GI tract, the more double-sugar intolerances and the more severe the symptoms. The most common disaccharidase deficiency is lactase, which breaks down lactose (cow's milk sugar) and is known as lactose intolerance.

More in-depth discussion of these treatments is beyond the scope of this book. For more information, refer to section 6.3 Specific Carbohydrate Diet (SCD) and Gut and Psychology Syndrome (GAPS) Diets. The following resources are available:
• *Breaking the Vicious Cycle* by Elaine Gottschall, www.breakingtheviciouscycle.info
• www.pecanbread.com
• *GAPS Gut and Psychology Syndrome* by Natasha Campbell-McBride, www.gapsdiet.com

What to Do and How to Do It
Treatment options include:
1. Avoidance of lactose-containing cow's milk products and other double sugar sources such as processed meats, beans, all grains, flours, potatoes, yams, dried fruits, canned vegetables, rice milk, and soy milk
2. Use of the SCD, which includes foods that do not have disaccharides (referred to as "SCD legal") foods:
   • Foods without starch/sugars: meat, seafood, poultry, eggs
   • Monosaccharide sugar/starch foods: nuts, vegetables, fruits, nut flours
   • Milk products and milk substitutes that are free of lactose and other disaccharides (double sugars)

Diarrhea

3. Use of digestive enzymes:
   - Lactase is the most common
   - Complete disaccharidase enzyme complex

What Enzymes Should I Use and Why?

Elimination diets are the most effective treatment. Enzymes are more helpful for small or hidden exposures.

Enzymes for lactose intolerance only: Lactaid is an over-the-counter supplement that provides the lactase enzyme. This can be taken at the beginning of a meal or snack that includes lactose-containing cow's milk products. Dosing may vary depending on the amount of cow's milk products ingested. For example, smaller amounts may require only one caplet while larger amounts may require two. Lactaid Original caplets contain mannitol, which is SCD illegal and can cause gas in some individuals. If this is problematic, consider using Lactaid Fast Act caplets, which do not contain mannitol. One Lactaid Fast Act caplet is equal to three Lactaid Original caplets.

ENZYMES FOR LACTOSE AND MILK INTOLERANCE ONLY

PRODUCT/ COMPANY	FUNCTION/ INFORMATION	SCD-COMPLIANT, GFCF*	AGE	PER MEAL
Lactaid Original 3,000 ALU/caplet	Lactase only Contains mannitol	GFCF only	2 to 5 6 to 10 11 +	½ to 1 caplet 1 to 2 caplets 2 to 3 caplets
Lactaid Fast Act caplets 9,000 ALU/caplet	Lactase only Contains no mannitol	Yes	2 to 5 6 to 10 11 +	⅓ caplet ⅓ to ⅔ caplet 1 caplet
BioCore Dairy made by *Kirkman* 1,000 ALU/capsule	Lactose and milk intolerance More effective than lactase alone.	Yes	2 to 5 6 to 10 11 +	1 caplet 1 to 2 caplets 2 to 3 caplets

*GLUTEN-FREE CASEIN-FREE

Enzymes for lactose and other disaccharide intolerance: The supplements include all of the disaccharidase enzymes: lactase, sucrose, maltase, isomaltase, and others.

ENZYMES FOR LACTOSE AND OTHER DISACCHARIDE INTOLERANCES

PRODUCT/COMPANY	FUNCTION/INFORMATION	SCD-COMPLIANT, GFCF*	AGE	PER MEAL
Carb Digest with Isogest, made by *Kirkman* 2,000 ALU/capsule	Disaccharidase enzymes for intolerance to double sugars	Yes	2 to 5 6 to 10 11 +	½ to 1 capsule 1 capsule 1 to 2 capsules
HN-Zyme Prime or Zyme Prime, made by *Houston Enzymes* 1,500 units/capsule	High lactase and other disaccharidase enzymes	Yes	2 to 5 6 to 10 11 +	½ to 1 capsule 1 capsule 1 to 2 capsules

- Enzymes are best taken at the beginning of the meal or snack. If the dose is delayed, enzymes can be given during the meal and up to one hour after the meal (the length of time it takes food to clear the stomach).
- The enzyme capsule/tablet can be swallowed or opened and the powder mixed into food or liquid.
- As soon as the enzyme mixes with food, it is active. Enzymes should therefore not be added into food or liquids and used at a later time.
- For a list of combination digestive enzymes for protein, fat, carbohydrates, lactose and other disaccharides, and opioid peptides, see the chart on page 231.

What Side Effects Should I Watch for?

In general, there are few side effects. It is possible that there could be some digestive distress; however, this is not common. The products are usually stool firming, which is most helpful with diarrhea.

Section D: Food Intolerances and Elimination of Opioid Food Culprits

Food intolerances can result in both behavioral and physical symptoms. Physical symptoms can include diarrhea because of motility problems, food reactions, food intolerances, and poor absorption of nutrients such as fats. A full discussion of food intolerances is beyond the scope of this book. More information and resources are available in section 4.17 Digestive Enzymes and section 6.1 Gluten-Free Casein-Free Soy-Free (GFCFSF) Diet.

What to Do and How to Do It

Provided here is a brief summary of two main treatment strategies for food intolerances and the opiate-like peptide effect.

1. GFCFSF Diet—Elimination Trial: the "gold standard" for treatment
   - The most common problem food proteins are gluten, milk casein, and soy.
   - Your child's body is the best test. Eliminate the food(s) to see whether behavior improves and reintroduce or challenge the body to see whether behavior worsens.
2. Digestive enzymes, including dipeptidyl peptidase-IV (DPP-IV)
   - More efficiently digest gluten, casein, soy and other food proteins, carbohydrates, and fats.
   - Reduce the opioid load due to insufficient DPP-IV enzyme function; this can also "mimic" the diet.

Digestive Enzyme Supplements

See section 4.17 Digestive Enzymes for detailed information on specific enzyme products and dosing.

Diarrhea

Section E: Treatment of Fat Malabsorption

Fat malabsorption can occur when fats are not digested adequately. Causes of fat malabsorption can include:

- Insufficient lipase, the main fat-digesting enzyme
- Insufficient or ineffective bile, a substance produced in the liver and released by the gallbladder
- Insufficient taurine, which is a component of bile
- Other medical conditions. If fat malabsorption is suspected, a medical workup by your child's primary care physician is indicated.

What to Do and How to Do it

If fat malabsorption is suspected, we recommend that your child have a medical evaluation by his or her primary care physician. Once that evaluation is completed, the following supplements may be considered, with your child's physician's knowledge.

Lipase is the main fat-digesting enzyme. The enzyme should be given at the beginning of the meal and not on an empty stomach.

LIPASE TOTAL DAILY GOAL DOSING

PRODUCT/COMPANY	DESCRIPTION	SCD-COMPLIANT, GFCF	AGE	PER MEAL
Lipase Concentrate-HP made by *Integrative Therapeutics*	Lipase I, II	GFCF-compliant	2 to 5 6 to 10 11 +	½ capsule 1 capsule 1 to 2 capsules

For a list of combination digestive enzymes for protein, fat (lipase), carbohydrates, lactose, other disaccharides, and opioid peptides, see section 4.17 Digestive Enzymes.

Taurine is a major component of bile and necessary for its effectiveness.

TAURINE TOTAL DAILY GOAL DOSING

AGE	DOSE	FREQUENCY	TOTAL DAILY DOSE FROM ALL SOURCES
2 to 5	150 mg	1 or 2 times per day	300 mg
6 to 10	150 mg	2 times per day	300 mg
11 +	250 mg	2 times per day	500 mg

The doses recommended are conservative. We would recommend the guidance of a health care practitioner when using taurine, especially if your child has an autism spectrum disorder. A subset of children with autism have metabolic disorders, some of which may render them intolerant to specific amino acids, including taurine. Starting with low doses will reveal any negative responses, which should resolve upon cessation. Blood and urine amino acid testing and a metabolic workup (to the degree determined necessary by a health care practitioner) will be helpful in guiding safe use of taurine.

What Else Should I Know?
There are several vitamins that are fat-soluble; they require fats to be absorbed in order to enter the body. These are vitamins A, D, E, and K. When fat malabsorption is present, these levels may be low. Blood testing can be done to determine these levels.

■ 2.8 Eye Contact and Vision Problems
Decreased eye contact is a common problem in children with autism. Nutrient deficiencies and sensory processing issues can both contribute to poor eye contact.

Symptoms/signs your child may exhibit
- Decreased eye contact: not looking when greeted or communicating, not using eye contact for social connection, and difficulty sustaining eye contact
- Increased use of peripheral vision or sideways glancing

Main possible contributing nutritional factors
- Omega-3 DHA and EPA deficiency
- Vitamin A deficiency
- Zinc deficiency
- Opioid peptides from gluten, milk casein, and possibly soy and corn

DETERMINING WHICH SUPPLEMENTS AND DIET CHANGES MAY BE HELPFUL

IF YOUR CHILD HAS POOR EYE CONTACT AND ONE OR MORE OF THE FOLLOWING SYMPTOMS	SEE THE APPLICABLE SECTION BELOW	DIETARY AND OTHER RECOMMENDATIONS	OTHER SOURCES OF INFORMATION
Cracking, peeling, chipping nails Attention problems Cognitive problems Language delays Eczema, dermatitis Excessive thirst Hard earwax	Section A: Essential Omega-3 Fatty Acids	Increase consumption of healthy omega-3 foods	Chapter 1: "Quick Start Diet" Chapter 4: section 4.15 Essential Omega-3 Fatty Acids
Night blindness Sideways glancing Frequent illness Eczema, dermatitis Keratosis pilaris (chicken skin)	Section B: Vitamin A		Chapter 4: section 4.1 Vitamin A

Eye Contact

Picky appetite White lines on nails Frequent illness Skin: Eczema, dermatitis Elevated toxic metals Developmental delays Growth delays Picky appetite Sensory sensitivities	Section C: Zinc		Chapter 4: section 4.9 Zinc
Food cravings for milk casein and/or gluten and/or soy In a "fog" or "own world" Bowel problems Unexplained laughing High pain tolerance Mood problems Cognitive problems Attention problems Language delays	Section D: Food Intolerances and Elimination of Opioid Food Culprits Digestive enzymes	Section D: Food Intolerances and Elimination of Opioid Food Culprits Gluten-Free Casein-Free Soy-Free (GFCFSF)	Chapter 4: section 4.17 Digestive Enzymes Chapter 6: section 6.1 GFCFSF Diet

Section A: Essential Omega-3 Fatty Acids

The essential omega-3 fatty acids are eicosapentaenoic acid (EPA) and docosahexaenoic acid (DHA). Almost 60 percent of the brain is composed of fat, with DHA being the primary structural component of the human brain and retina. DHA also affects focus and attention.

What to Do and How to Do It

Provided here is a brief summary on omega-3 fatty acids. For thorough information and specific guidelines on supplement brands, dosing, and side effects, see section 4.15 Essential Omega-3 Fatty Acids.

The best food sources of omega-3 fatty acids are seafood. Those highest in mercury, PCBs, and other toxins include tomally (crab mustard), farmed fish, trout, imported shrimp, and the large "steak" fish such as tuna, bluefish, swordfish, and shark. The safest choices include anchovies, sardines, domestic shrimp, rockfish, and tilapia. For details, see the Environmental Working Group website, www.ewg.org, and the Environmental Defense Fund website, www.edf.org.

Omega-3 supplements
- For vision as well as focus, attention, and cognition, we recommend that DHA amount be equal to or greater than the EPA.
- Use only direct source EPA and DHA, which is more efficient than flaxseed source ALA.
- Use toxin-free supplements: pharmaceutical grade or molecular distillation to remove toxins.

Types of high DHA omega-3 supplements available in capsules, liquids, and chewables
- Cod liver oil (contains varying amounts of vitamins A and D)
- Fish oils with increased DHA to EPA ratio
- Vegetarian algae-source DHA

The following supplements have substantial levels of DHA:
- Barleans Omega Swirl
- Omega Cure (unflavored)
- Nordic Naturals ProOmega or Ultimate Omega
- Carlson Norwegian Cod Liver Oil with A and D$_3$
- Genestra Super DHA Liquid
- Nordic Naturals Baby's DHA (and EPA)
- Neuromins DHA caps (algae-source DHA)
- Nordic Naturals ProDHA 1,000 soft gels

OMEGA-3 EPA AND DHA TOTAL DAILY GOAL DOSING

AGE	EPA	DHA	FREQUENCY
2 to 5	200 to 400 mg	200 to 400 mg	Daily with food
6 to 10	500 to 650 mg	400 to 500 mg	Daily with food
11 +	500 to 800 mg	500 to 650 mg	Daily with food

- Though DHA is preferred for assisting in eye contact, attention, focus, communication, and mood, EPA is also important and should be included.
- Higher-than-recommended doses of omega-3 fatty acids should only be given under the guidance of a skilled health care practitioner.

Section B: Vitamin A

A subset of children with autism has vitamin A deficiency. Vitamin A is a fat-soluble vitamin, critical for vision, especially night vision. When the retina of the eye is deprived of vitamin A, rod and cone function is impaired. Although we do not fully understand how vitamin A affects eye contact, the clinical experience is impressive. When vitamin A deficiency is a significant factor, improvements in eye contact may be seen within weeks of adequate supplementation. The sideways glancing declines or resolves and the child makes direct eye contact without prompting.

What to Do and How to Do It
Provided here is a brief summary on vitamin A. For thorough information and specific guidelines on dosing and side effects, see section 4.1 Vitamin A.

To ensure adequate vitamin A, include preformed vitamin A that is found in animal sources and synthesized. Beta-carotene converts to vitamin A and is not recommended as the main treatment for vitamin A deficiency. The conversion of beta-carotene to vitamin A may not be efficient in some individuals. Giving preformed vitamin A is recommended.

Vitamin A supplements
- Preformed vitamin A is more effective and is found in the following types:
  - Retinoids
  - Micellized vitamin A (water-soluble, well-absorbed form)
- Synthetic vitamin A palmitate

Eye Contact

VITAMIN A TOTAL DAILY GOAL DOSING

AGE	DAILY DOSE FROM ALL SOURCES
2 to 3	1,250 IU
4 to 5	1,250 to 2,500 IU
6 to 10	2,500 to 3,500 IU
11 +	3,500 to 5,000 IU

- Micellized vitamin products are absorbed more efficiently and are useful in poor absorption conditions.
- Commercially available micellized vitamin A products are usually high dose (5,000 IU). More appropriate strength drops can be made by a compounding pharmacy.
- Zinc is critical for vitamin A transport and utilization. See section C.
- Excess vitamin A can result in headaches.
- Higher doses may be required because of poor absorption or lab findings. This should be accomplished with a skilled health care practitioner.
- Adequate vitamin D is required when taking vitamin A.

VITAMIN D TOTAL DAILY GOAL DOSING

AGE	DOSE	FREQUENCY
2 to 5	400 to 600 IU	Daily
6 to 10	600 to 800 IU	Daily
11 +	800 to 2,000 IU	Daily

Section C: Zinc

Zinc is critical to vitamin A, which is carried in the body by zinc-dependent retinol-binding protein. When zinc is deficient (and therefore vitamin A as well), eye contact can suffer. Zinc deficiency is extremely common in children with autism and is not unusual in children with ADHD.

What to Do and How to Do It

Provided here is a brief summary on zinc. For thorough information and specific guidelines on dosing and side effects, see section 4.9 Zinc.

Zinc supplements
- Well-tolerated forms: gluconates, chelates, citrates, acetates, picolinates, chlorides, and bisglycinates
- Form that has a strong taste, which needs disguising: sulfates

ZINC TOTAL DAILY GOAL DOSING

AGE	DOSE	FREQUENCY	TOTAL DAILY DOSE FROM ALL SOURCES
2 to 5	5 to 10 mg	1 or 2 times per day	10 to 20 mg
6 to 10	10 mg	2 times per day	20 mg
11 +	10 to 15 mg	2 times per day	20 to 30 mg

For optimal oral absorption, an empty stomach is best, but it may not be feasible if nausea occurs. Large doses can cause gastric discomfort, nausea, and inhibit the digestive enzyme DPP-IV (digests opioids from gluten, casein). In addition:

- Avoid or limit giving zinc at the same time as interfering nutrients: calcium, iron, folate, and phosphorylated nutrients (R5P, P5P, phosphatidyl-choline); this may not always be feasible.
- Zinc excess can lower copper. Copper levels need to be maintained.
- Use the Zinc Tally Taste Test on page 213 for evaluating progress with zinc supplementation.
- Higher doses may be required due to poor absorption, antacid use, toxic metals, or lab findings. This should be accomplished with the help of a skilled health care practitioner.

Section D: Food Intolerances and Elimination of Opioid Food Culprits

A common effect of food intolerance is poor eye contact. A full discussion of food intolerances is beyond the scope of this book. More information and resources are available in section 4.17 Digestive Enzymes and section 6.1 Gluten-Free Casein-Free Soy-Free (GFCFSF) Diet.

In short, food proteins, particularly those from milk (casein) and wheat (gluten), may be incompletely digested to peptides and may enter the bloodstream from the intestine via an abnormally permeable intestinal lining (referred to as "leaky gut"). These partially digested protein peptides can potentially cross the blood–brain barrier, negatively affecting brain function, including contributing to mood, attention, and behavior by several mechanisms:

- Blocking neurotransmitter messages
- Creating opiate-like doping effects from gluten (gliadorphin), milk casein (casomorphin), and soy
- Triggering brain inflammation

The most obvious symptom is a craving for the food opiate sources (gluten, milk products, and soy). In addition to poor eye contact, other symptoms include inattention, poor focus, language delays, irritability, and increased activity and repeated self-stimulatory behaviors. Effects may occur within an hour of consumption or be delayed up to seventy-two hours.

What to Do and How to Do It
Provided on the next page is a brief summary of two main treatment strategies for food intolerances and the opioid effect.

Eye Contact

1. GFCFSF Diet—Elimination Trial: the "gold standard" for treatment
   - The most common problem food proteins are gluten, milk casein, and soy.
   - Your child's body is the best test. Eliminate the food(s) to see whether behavior improves and reintroduce or challenge the body to see whether behavior worsens.
2. Digestive enzymes, including dipeptidyl peptidase-IV (DPP-IV)
   - More efficiently digest gluten, casein, soy and other food proteins, carbohydrates, and fats.
   - Reduce the opioid load due to insufficient DPP-IV enzyme function; this can also "mimic" the diet.

Digestive Enzyme Supplements
See section 4.17 Digestive Enzymes for detailed information on specific enzyme products and dosing.

■ 2.9 Fatigue, Poor Endurance, and Low Muscle Tone

Fatigue or poor endurance can stem from a number of factors and affect attention and availability for learning. Low muscle tone can result in reduced ability to participate in normal gross motor play and social activities such as sports.

Symptoms/signs your child may exhibit
- Decreased stamina, tiring out before other children
- Exercise intolerance
- Unusual fatigue
- Low muscle tone

Main possible contributing factors
- Magnesium deficiency
- Iron deficiency
- Zinc deficiency
- Carnitine deficiency
- Need for coenzyme Q_{10} (CoQ_{10})
- B vitamin deficiencies: B_6, B_{12}, folate

DETERMINING WHICH SUPPLEMENTS AND DIET CHANGES MAY BE HELPFUL

IF YOUR CHILD HAS FATIGUE, POOR ENDURANCE AND SOME OF THE FOLLOWING SYMPTOMS	SEE THE APPLICABLE SECTION BELOW	DIETARY AND OTHER RECOMMENDATIONS	OTHER SOURCES OF INFORMATION
Constipation Sound sensitivity Easy to startle Anxiety Mood swings Sleep disruption Excessive sighing Muscle spasms	Section A: Magnesium	Higher intake of magnesium-rich foods: vegetables, beans, nuts, seeds, fruits	Chapter 4: section 4.8 Magnesium and Calcium

Decreased energy Pale skin Pallor inside lower eyelid Nail-bed pallor upon pressure Dizzy upon standing Craving for chewing ice	Section B: Iron	Red meat, chicken, seafood, beans, nuts, seeds	
Picky appetite White lines on nails Frequent illness Skin problems	Section C: Zinc		Chapter 4: section 4.9 Zinc
Tongue: Fissures Redness Geographic (migrans) Soreness Angular cheilosis (cracks in corner of mouth)	Section D: B Vitamins		Chapter 4: sections 4.4 and 4.5 on B vitamins
Weak muscles No red meat in diet Vegan diet	Section E: Carnitine	Red meat	Chapter 4: section 4.13 Carnitine
Weak muscles Shortness of breath Low-fat diet Fat malabsorption Use of beta-blocker and/or statin medications	Section F: CoQ_{10}		Chapter 4: section 4.14 Coenzyme Q_{10}
Low muscle tone	Section G: Physical and/or Occupational Therapy	Optimal protein intake	Chapter 4: sections 4.4, 4.5, 4.9, 4.13, and 4.14

Fatigue

Section A: Magnesium

Magnesium is critical in energy metabolism, especially adenosine triphosphate (ATP), which is the body's energy molecule, produced in the mitochondria (furnace of the cell). Low magnesium levels impair the efficiency of muscle contraction and relaxation leading to elevated lactic acid, which causes poor muscle endurance. Magnesium deficiency causes poor protein utilization, which also affects muscle strength and endurance.

What To Do and How to Do It

Provided here is a brief summary on magnesium. For thorough information and specific guidelines on dosing and side effects, see section 4.8 Magnesium and Calcium.

  Magnesium supplements

- Gentle (less laxative) stool effect: chelates, aspartates, glycinates, gluconates, and bisglycinates
- Laxative stool effect: citrates, chlorides, sulfates

MAGNESIUM TOTAL DAILY GOAL DOSING

AGE	DOSE	FREQUENCY	TOTAL DAILY DOSE FROM ALL SOURCES
2 to 5	100 mg	1 or 2 times per day	200 mg
6 to 10	100 mg	2 or 3 times per day	300 mg
11 +	100 to 150 mg	2 or 3 times per day	450 mg

- Start at one-quarter to one-half of the recommended dose and increase the dose gradually every one to two days.
- Magnesium can cause loose stools or diarrhea.
- Watch for possible side effects and decrease the dose accordingly.
- If symptoms improve at lower than the goal dose, you may not need to continue to increase the dose.
- For higher-than-recommended doses, consult with a health care practitioner.

Calcium
Make sure calcium intake, either through diet or supplementation, is adequate. Magnesium intake can lower calcium and calcium intake can lower magnesium. It is important to have balance. If your child is not getting sufficient calcium from diet, a calcium supplement is indicated.

CALCIUM TOTAL DAILY GOAL DOSING

AGE	DOSE	FREQUENCY	TOTAL DAILY DOSE FROM ALL SOURCES
2 to 5	250 mg	2 times per day	500 mg
6 to 10	250 mg	3 times per day	750 mg
11 +	500 to 600 mg	2 times per day	1,000 to 1,200 mg

Section B: Iron
Iron is responsible for oxygen delivery to the tissues. Muscle endurance is iron-dependent. Iron is also an important cofactor in carnitine production (see section E). Deficiencies of iron occur in both autism and ADHD.

Body stores of iron, as shown by low ferritin levels in blood testing, decline first, prior to serum iron declining. These deficits occur before the complete blood count indicates anemia. For this reason, inattention, poor endurance, lethargy, or fatigue may show up before the complete blood count reveals there is a problem.

What to Do and How to Do It
Provided here is a brief summary on iron. For more information, see the section on iron in chapter 4. Iron should never be given without blood testing to document whether your child has a need for iron. If levels of iron are too high or there is a metabolic disorder in which iron accumulates in the tissues, iron

supplementation can be damaging and even toxic. Consider these tests to determine levels: complete blood count, serum iron, TIBC, percent saturation, and serum ferritin (a measure of iron stores). When taking iron, routine follow-up blood testing is critical.

Iron dietary sources
- The richest and best-absorbed iron (heme)—is found in meats, especially liver.
- Plant sources of iron (nonheme) are less well absorbed (beans, nuts, seeds, and spinach).

Iron supplements
- All forms of iron supplements can darken the stool (depending upon the dose).
- Iron supplements can cause constipation, especially the sulfate forms.
- Forms that are well tolerated by the digestive tract are: ferrous fumarate, gluconate, chelates, and bisglycinate.

IRON TOTAL DAILY GOAL DOSING

AGE	DOSE	FREQUENCY	TOTAL DAILY DOSE FROM ALL SOURCES
2 to 5	7 to 10 mg	Daily	7 to 10 mg
6 to 10	10 mg	Daily	10 mg
11 +	8 to 10 mg	Daily	8 to 10 mg

- We strongly recommend that you do not give iron for the treatment of fatigue and poor endurance without consulting with a physician and having appropriate blood testing. Dosing based on blood testing may be significantly different from the amounts listed in the chart.
- Iron is best taken at a different time from calcium, zinc, phosphorus, fiber, and vitamin E.
- The main side effect of treatment with iron is constipation, which can be resolved by adding magnesium and/or vitamin C. See section 2.6 Constipation.

Copper's Role in Anemia
Copper is important for hemoglobin metabolism, low levels of which can cause microcytic anemia, which looks like iron deficiency but is not responsive to iron. Because elevated copper is more common than copper deficiency in ADHD and autism, copper supplementation is not recommended without testing for copper.

Section C: Zinc
Zinc is necessary for the utilization of amino acids, which the body needs to build muscle. Muscle development and tone also depend upon excellent intake of protein, which is then digested into amino acids, absorbed, and transported to the cells for use.

Fatigue

Zinc deficiency can limit amino acid metabolism by the cells. Even if there is good protein intake, if zinc is deficient, the effect is the same as low protein intake and low amino acid availability.

What to Do and How to Do It
Provided here is a brief summary on zinc. For more information, see section 4.9.

Zinc supplements
- Well tolerated: gluconates, chelates, citrates, acetates, picolinates, chlorides, and bisglycinates
- Strong taste, needs disguising: sulfates

ZINC TOTAL DAILY GOAL DOSING

AGE	DOSE	FREQUENCY	TOTAL DAILY DOSE FROM ALL SOURCES
2 to 5	5 to 10 mg	1 or 2 times per day	10 to 20 mg
6 to 10	10 mg	2 times per day	20 mg
11 +	10 to 15 mg	2 times per day	20 to 30 mg

For optimal oral absorption, an empty stomach is best, but it may not be feasible if nausea occurs. Large doses can cause gastric discomfort, nausea, and inhibit the digestive enzyme DPP-IV (digests opioids from gluten and casein). In addition:
- Avoid or limit giving zinc at the same time as interfering nutrients: calcium, iron, folate, and phosphorylated nutrients (R5P, P5P, phosphatidyl-choline), although this may not always be feasible.
- Zinc excess can lower copper. Copper levels need to be maintained.
- If not able to get blood tests, use the Zinc Tally Taste test on page 213 for evaluating progress with zinc supplementation.
- Higher doses may be required because of poor absorption, antacid use, toxic metals, or lab findings. This should be accomplished with the help of a skilled health care practitioner.

Section D: B Vitamins
B vitamins are water-soluble and critical in cellular energy metabolism pathways.

There is an interdependence among the B vitamins. For this reason, we usually recommend a B vitamin complex (separately or as part of a multiple vitamin–mineral), with the option to add additional individual B vitamins as indicated by symptoms and/or lab findings.

Fatigue and poor endurance are common in B vitamin deficiencies, particularly deficiencies of B_6 (pyridoxine), B_{12} (methylcobalamin), and folinic acid. All three support methylation, which is important in neurotransmitters, gene expression, cell membranes, and DNA. Methylation is defective in many of those with autism as well as some children with ADHD. A gene mutation—MTHFR (methylenetetrahydrofolate reductase) defect—renders the individual dependent on therapeutic doses of the methylation nutrients.

What to Do and How to Do It

Provided here is a brief summary on B_6, B_{12}, and folinic acid. For thorough information and specific guidelines on dosing and side effects, see section 4.5 Methylation Nutrients.

In fatigue, there are two primary types of anemia that involve B vitamins:

- Macrocytic, which is most responsive to B_{12} and folic acid
- Microcytic, which is most responsive to iron, copper, and/or B_6

Testing for anemia and deficiencies of B_6, B_{12}, and folinic acid should be accomplished by a skilled health care practitioner. Blood tests for serum iron and ferritin are reliable indicators of iron deficiency. However, serum levels of the B vitamins are not sensitive markers for deficiency and do not decline until extreme late stages of deficiency. There are metabolite tests that are more specific for B vitamin functional status.

Supplements

Multiple vitamin and B complex supplements may or may not have sufficient levels of these B vitamins. Added doses may be required.

Vitamin B_6
- Pyridoxal-5′-phosphate is the active cofactor form.
- B_6 is more effective if taken with magnesium.
- If sulfation (involved in detoxification, immunity, neurotransmitters, and energy metabolism) is defective, as is the case with phenol sensitivities/intolerances, avoid the pyridoxal-5′-phosphate form of B_6 supplements.

VITAMIN B_6 TOTAL DAILY GOAL DOSING

AGE	DOSE
2 to 5	15 mg
6 to 10	30 mg
11 +	50 mg

Vitamin B_{12}
- Methylcobalamin and hydroxocobalamin are active forms with excellent bioavailability.
- Poor absorption and/or the use of antacids can cause B_{12} deficiency.
- Sublingual forms may be preferred (they bypass the stomach).

VITAMIN B_{12} TOTAL DAILY GOAL DOSING

AGE	DOSE
2 to 5	100 mcg
6 to 10	500 mcg
11 +	1,000 mcg

Fatigue

Folinic acid
- Folinic acid is one of the preferred folate forms noted for its excellent bioavailability.
- Folic acid is least effective and best avoided.
- Absorption can be hindered by antacids, antiseizure medications, and tetracycline.

FOLINIC ACID TOTAL DAILY GOAL DOSING

AGE	DOSE
2 to 5	100 mcg
6 to 10	200 mcg
11 +	500 mcg

Side effects of any one or all of these nutrients can include increased activity, stimming, irritability, or anxiety. If these symptoms occur, stop the supplement and discuss with your health care practitioner.

Section E: Carnitine
Carnitine is synthesized in the body from the amino acids lysine and methionine. L-carnitine, a biologically active form of carnitine, helps the body turn fat into energy. It is required for the transport of long chain fatty acids into the mitochondria, the energy-generating machinery in cells. Low levels can result in poor endurance, weak muscles (including weak cardiac muscles), or fatigue. Potential causes of carnitine deficiency include:
- Poor intake of red meat, the main dietary source of carnitine. Children on vegetarian diets and with picky appetites are at risk for carnitine deficiency.
- Deficiencies of iron, B vitamins, lysine, methionine, and vitamin C.
- Use of certain seizure medications that can lower carnitine.
- Metabolic/mitochondrial disorders. While severe metabolic disorders are uncommon, metabolic dysfunction or milder forms of metabolic disorders are now known to occur in a subset of children with autism.

There are rare metabolic disorders (LCHAD, VLCAD) that can include cardiomyopathy (a weakening of the heart muscle). In these conditions, L-carnitine may cause abnormal heart rhythms. It can also aggravate seizures in certain susceptible individuals. Cardiomyopathy can occur when carnitine levels are very low; hence, blood testing is important before L-carnitine is used.

What to Do and How to Do It
There are two primary forms of carnitine supplements: L-carnitine and acetyl-L-carnitine. L-carnitine is recommended when treating general symptoms such as fatigue or poor endurance. Acetyl-L-carnitine may be more helpful for supporting brain function.

The D and DL forms of carnitine should be avoided. They are not functional and can cause serious problems.

Lower doses of carnitine are used to treat dietary causes of low carnitine while much higher doses may be needed to treat metabolic dysfunctions or inefficiencies.

How Do I Dose Carnitine?
Because of the possibility of potential problems, L-carnitine supplementation is not recommended without blood testing. Supplementation should be accomplished only under the care of a knowledgeable health care practitioner who can determine whether additional testing is indicated before carnitine use.

Dosing of carnitine is dependent on the cause of the low carnitine as well as the blood level.

What Side Effects Should I Watch for?
Some children may have a worsening of behavior on L-carnitine, as a direct side effect or due to the body adjusting to increased energy and alertness from carnitine. Loose stools are also possible. At high doses, carnitine can result in a fishy body smell.

What Else Should I Know?
Clues to metabolic disorders can include:
- Unusual lethargy with illnesses or fasting
- Loss of skills in association with illnesses
- Unusual odor in urine or sweat
- Unusual food aversions, such as avoidance of all proteins or all sweet foods

If your child has these symptoms, please discuss them with his or her primary care provider.

Section F: Coenzyme Q_{10}
Coenzyme Q_{10} (CoQ_{10}) is a fat-soluble compound synthesized in the body and also available to a limited degree in the diet. It is a ubiquinone named for its ubiquitous presence in living organisms. CoQ_{10} in the cell mitochondrial membrane converts energy from carbohydrates and fats to adenosine triphosphate, the form of energy used by the body.

CoQ_{10} is responsible for 95 percent of the energy produced for the body. If there is deficiency in the enzyme or its function, the body experiences a "brown out" during which there is not sufficient energy to accomplish all its functions. The result is fatigue, poor endurance, lethargy, and muscle weakness.

In addition to energy metabolism, CoQ_{10} functions as an antioxidant, and is important in gene expression, immunity, cardiovascular function, muscle function, and neurological function.

Our recommendations here are focused on mitochondrial inefficiencies or dysfunctions, not the serious, life-threatening mitochondrial diseases. There is a subset of children with autism who have these lesser inefficiencies/dysfunctions, which can be responsive to treatment.

Urinary metabolite testing can identify inefficiencies in function, and guide treatment. There are blood tests and also muscle biopsies for the more serious presentations.

What to Do and How to Do It
There are various forms of CoQ_{10} supplements
- Compared to dry powder forms, oil-based emulsion soft gels have better absorption and bioavailability.
- Liquid forms are available:
Life Time CoQ_{10} liquid 1 tsp = 50 mg
NOW Liquid CoQ_{10} 1 tsp = 100 mg
- CoQ_{10} as ubiquinone converts to ubinquinol, the active form, for function.

There are a few studies showing the ubiquinol form to be better in absorption and bioavailability.
- If taking a dry form of CoQ_{10}, taking it with a fatty meal will improve absorption and bioavailability.

COQ_{10} TOTAL DAILY GOAL DOSING

AGE	DOSE	TOTAL DAILY DOSE FROM ALL SOURCES
2 to 5	25 to 50 mg	25 to 50 mg
6 to 10	50 to 75 mg	50 to 75 mg
11 +	100 mg	100 mg

CoQ_{10} supplements are considered safe, and no RDA or toxic dose has been identified. For higher doses, consult a health care practitioner.

What Side Effects Should I Watch for?
Digestive symptoms can occur with intakes above 3,000 mg.

What Else Should I Know?
- Cholesterol-lowering medications known as statin drugs and beta-blockers used for lowering blood pressure can lower body stores of CoQ_{10}.
- Higher doses of CoQ_{10} can decrease the effectiveness of blood-thinning medications such as warfarin and tricyclic antidepressant medications.

Section G: Physical and/or Occupational Therapy
Muscle tone refers to the amount of tension or resistance to movement in a muscle. Tone can be high, as seen in individuals with spasticity (such as in some forms of cerebral palsy). Muscle tone can also be low, as seen in various neurological, muscle, or genetic disorders. It is also a common finding to some degree in children with behavioral or developmental issues. Muscle tone helps in maintaining body posture. When tone is low, it requires more muscle strength to compensate. For example, when tone is low through the trunk, it requires more core muscle strength to maintain an upright position. If low tone is significant, it can affect endurance.

Signs of low muscle tone may include:
- Hypermobile joints at fingers, knees, elbows
- General "floppy" appearance
- Difficulty maintaining upright posture; tendency to slouch when sitting
- Preference to sit with legs in a "W" position

What to Do and How to Do It
The main treatment for low muscle tone is therapy with an occupational or physical therapist to maximize both strength and sensory regulation. The effectiveness of therapies can be limited by the muscle's ability to receive the nutrients necessary for healthy muscle function. With deficiencies in a specific set of nutrients, the tissues can become oxygen starved and take much longer to recover. Mitochondrial inefficiencies may also be present.

Specific supplements may help improve tone by improving core energy (mitochondrial) metabolism and amino acid utilization. (Amino acids are the building blocks of protein, which is important for building muscle.)

What Supplements Should I Use and Why?
Many nutrients and cofactors are involved in energy metabolism. The following are the most important; the prior sections in this chapter explain the rationale for their use:

- Magnesium
- Iron
- L-carnitine
- Coenzyme Q_{10}
- B vitamins
- Biotin

Amino acid metabolism and utilization is supported primarily by zinc and vitamin B_6. If your child's protein intake is insufficient, increased dietary protein or amino acid supplements may be indicated.

What Else Should I Know?
Prior to considering using a general amino acid supplement, we would recommend blood testing for amino acids. For children with autism, additional evaluation for possible metabolic disorders may also be indicated prior to using amino acid supplements.

■ *2.10 Hyperactivity*
Hyperactivity is an important symptom in two subtypes of ADHD. It is also commonly seen in children with autism. Hyperactivity can interfere with both academic and social learning.

Symptoms/signs your child may exhibit
- Above-average activity level
- Frequent movement, including "fidgetiness"
- Difficulty staying seated in class
- Distractibility

- Difficulty staying on task
- Boundary issues, including invading others' personal space and talking too loudly
- Impulsivity
- Tossing and turning during sleep

Main possible contributing nutritional factors:
- Magnesium deficiency
- Omega-3 fatty acid deficiency
- Sensitivity to synthetic food additives, coloring, and flavoring
- Sensitivity to phenols and need for taurine
- Excess glutamate and need for GABA and vitamin B_6
- Food intolerances (e.g., casein, gluten, soy)

DETERMINING WHICH SUPPLEMENTS AND DIET CHANGES MAY BE HELPFUL

IF YOUR CHILD HAS HYPERACTIVITY AND SOME OF THE FOLLOWING SYMPTOMS	SEE THE APPLICABLE SECTION BELOW	DIETARY AND OTHER RECOMMENDATIONS	OTHER SOURCES OF INFORMATION
Constipation Sound sensitivity Easy startle Anxiety Mood swings Sleep disruption Excessive sighing Poor muscle endurance	Section A: Magnesium	Higher intake of magnesium-rich foods: vegetables, beans, nuts, seeds, fruits	Chapter 4, section 4.8 Magnesium and Calcium
Cracking, peeling, chipping nails Attention problems Cognitive problems Language delays Vision dysfunction Eczema, dermatitis Excessive thirst Hard earwax	Section B: Essential Omega-3 Fatty Acids	Increase consumption of healthy omega-3 foods	Chapter 4: section 4.15 Essential Omega-3 Fatty Acids
Immediate increase in hyperactivity, fidgeting, and distractibility after consumption of foods with artificial additives, coloring, flavoring	Section C: Organic Diet Free of Artificial Additives	Section C: Organic Diet Free of Artificial Additives	Chapter 1: "Quick Start Diet" Chapter 6: section 6.2 Low Phenol Diet
Red cheeks or ears without obvious explanation Sweating at night Difficulty sleeping Unexplained giggling	Section D: Phenol Sensitivity	Section D: Phenol Sensitivity	Chapter 4: section 4.8 Magnesium and Calcium Chapter 6: section 6.2 Low Phenol Diet
Anxiety Obsessive–compulsive symptoms Language delay Sleep problems	Section E: High Glutamate and Need for GABA and Vitamin B_6	Section E: High Glutamate and Need for GABA and Vitamin B_6 Limit/avoid glutamate (excitotoxins): MSG, milk products, gluten, aspartame	Chapter 4: section 4.11 GABA and Theanine and section 4.5 Vitamin B_6 Chapter 6: section 6.2 Low Phenol Diet

| Food cravings for milk casein and/or gluten and/or soy In a "fog" or "own world" Bowel problems Unexplained laughing High pain tolerance Poor eye contact Mood problems Attention problems Language delays | Section F: Food Intolerances and Elimination of Opioid Food Culprits | Section F: Food Intolerances and Elimination of Opioid Food Culprits Gluten-Free Casein-Free Soy-Free (GFCFSF) diet | Chapter 4: section 4.17 Digestive Enzymes Chapter 6: section 6.1 GFCFSF Diet |

Hyperactivity

Section A: Magnesium

Magnesium is a common nutritional deficiency in children with ADHD or autism. It is also a common deficiency in the general population. Low levels of magnesium result in neuromuscular excitability, which leads to increased activity and movement, distractibility, impulsivity, attention problems, and difficulty staying still. Magnesium is calming neurologically, which reduces hyperactivity and also improves attention, focus, sleep, and endurance in addition to reducing constipation, sound sensitivity, anxiety, and mood swings.

Taurine improves magnesium function and has an overall calming effect on the nervous system.

What to Do and How to Do It

Provided here is a brief summary on magnesium. For thorough information and specific guidelines on dosing and side effects, see section 4.8 Magnesium and Calcium and section 4.12 Taurine.

Magnesium supplements
- Gentle (less laxative) stool effect: chelates, aspartates, glycinates, gluconates, and bisglycinates
- Laxative stool effect: citrates, chlorides, and sulfates

MAGNESIUM TOTAL DAILY GOAL DOSING

AGE	DOSE	FREQUENCY	TOTAL DAILY DOSE FROM ALL SOURCES
2 to 5	100 mg	1 or 2 times per day	200 mg
6 to 10	100 mg	2 or 3 times per day	300 mg
11 +	100 to 150 mg	2 or 3 times per day	450 mg

- Start at one-quarter to one-half of the recommended dose and increase the dose gradually every one to two days.
- Magnesium can cause loose stools or diarrhea.
- Watch for possible side effects and decrease the dose accordingly.
- If symptoms improve at lower than the goal dose, you may not need to continue to increase the dose.
- For higher than recommended doses, consult with a health care practitioner.

Calcium intake should be adequate when taking magnesium. Excess magnesium intake can lower calcium, and excess calcium intake can lower magnesium. It is important to have balance. If your child is not getting sufficient calcium from diet, a calcium supplement is indicated.

Section B: Essential Omega-3 Fatty Acids

The essential omega-3 fatty acids are eicosapenaenoic acid (EPA) and docosahexaenoic acid (DHA). Almost 60 percent of the brain is composed of fat, with DHA being the primary structural component of the human brain and retina. DHA also affects behavior, focus, and attention.

What to Do and How to Do It

Provided here is a brief summary on omega-3 fatty acids. For thorough information and specific guidelines on supplement brands, dosing, and side effects, see section 4.15 Essential Omega-3 Fatty Acids.

The best food sources of omega-3 fatty acids are found in seafood. Those highest in mercury, PCBs, and other toxins include tomalley (crab mustard), farmed fish trout, imported shrimp, and the large "steak" fish such as tuna, bluefish, swordfish, and shark. The safest choices include anchovies, sardines, domestic shrimp, rockfish, and tilapia. For details, see the Environmental Working Group website, www.ewg.org, and the Environmental Defense Fund website, www.edf.org.

Omega-3 supplements for hyperactivity
- The DHA amount should be equal to or greater than the EPA.
- Use only direct-source EPA and DHA, which is more efficient than the flaxseed-source ALA.
- Use toxin-free supplements: pharmaceutical grade or molecular distillation to remove toxins.

Types of omega-3 supplements available in capsules, liquids, and chewables:
- Cod liver oil (contains varying amounts of vitamins A and D)
- Fish oils with increased DHA-to-EPA ratio
- Vegetarian algae-source DHA

The following supplements have substantial levels of DHA. See section 4.15 Essential Omega-3 Fatty Acids for a complete listing of specific omega-3 supplements.
- Barleans Omega Swirl
- Omega Cure (unflavored)
- Nordic Naturals ProOmega or Ultimate Omega
- Carlson Norwegian Cod Liver Oil with A and D_3
- Genestra Super DHA Liquid
- Nordic Naturals Baby's DHA (and EPA)
- Neuromins DHA caps (algae source DHA)
- Nordic Naturals ProDHA 1,000 soft gels

OMEGA-3 EPA AND DHA TOTAL DAILY GOAL DOSING

AGE	EPA	DHA	FREQUENCY
2 to 5	200 to 400 mg	200 to 400 mg	Daily with food
6 to 10	500 to 650 mg	400 to 500 mg	Daily with food
11 +	500 to 800 mg	500 to 650 mg	Daily with food

- While DHA is most important for behavior, EPA is also important, and a combination product is preferred when possible.
- Higher doses of omega-3 fatty acids should only be given under the guidance of a skilled health care practitioner.

If using cod liver oil as the DHA source, make sure that the vitamin A content from cod liver oil, the multiple vitamin mineral supplement, and additional vitamin A do not exceed the doses on page 175.

Section C: Organic Diet Free of Artificial Additives

Food additives may also result in hyperactivity and sensitivities. Common offending agents include artificial additives, preservatives, flavoring, coloring, sweeteners, glutamates, and salicylates (a subset of phenols), including foods, aspirin, and aspirin-containing medications.

Based on a British study reporting that food colorings and/or sodium benzoate increase hyperactive behavior in children (2007, *The Lancet*), the American Academy of Pediatrics has acknowledged that a "low-additive diet is a valid intervention for children with ADHD" (AAP Grand Rounds, Feb 2008). Some children may need to strictly remove the majority of these offending agents while others improve from decreasing the amount. Two diets are the low phenol/low salicylate diet (Feingold diet) and, the most comprehensive, the Failsafe diet.

Section D: Phenol Sensitivity

Phenols are naturally occurring beneficial nutritional chemicals found in high concentration in a variety of foods, especially cow's milk products, apples, bananas, red grapes, berries, and tomatoes. The enzyme, phenol sulfotransferase (PST), uses sulfate to metabolize phenols. When PST and/or sulfate is deficient, phenols fail to be metabolized well and sensitivity occurs. For a subset of children, especially those with autism, sulfate levels are inadequate.

- Aspirin, and artificial food additives, coloring, and flavorings are the most significant load on the PST system.
- Excess B_6 as pyridoxal-5'-phosphate can inhibit the enzyme and its functioning.
- Symptoms of phenol sensitivity include hyperactivity, red cheeks or red ears without an obvious explanation, night sweating, poor sleep, and/or unexplained giggling or silliness.

Hyperactivity

What to Do and How to Do It
There are three treatment options for treating phenol sensitivity:
- Use of sulfate to help the PST enzyme work better
- Removal of items with the highest phenol content: all synthetic additives in the diet, and medications (after consulation with a health care practitioner)
- Limiting of foods with high phenol content

How to Provide Sulfate
Sulfate improves PST enzyme function and enhances detoxification. The following three strategies should be helpful:
1. Magnesium sulfate topical lotion
   - Magnesium sulfate lotion 100 mg dose per gram of cream (Kirkman Labs)
   - Apply lotion to muscle areas in which absorption is highest: shoulders, back, or calves.
   - Massage in thoroughly. It may take 30 minutes to absorb, after which other lotions can be applied.
   - Rotate the application sites to reduce skin irritation.
   - If skin irritation or rash occurs, consider a custom compounded hypoallergenic lotion.
   - Topical magnesium sulfate lotion is not a good source of magnesium.

MAGNESIUM SULFATE TOPICAL LOTION TOTAL DAILY GOAL DOSING

DOSE
Starting dose: 100 mg in the morning
After 2 to 3 days: 100 mg morning and evening
After 2 to 3 more days: 100 mg morning, noon (or after school), and evening

2. Epsom salts and baking soda baths
   - To a bath of tolerated hot water add:
     —Epsom salt: 1 to 2 cups
     —Bicarbonate: 1 to 2 cups
   - Stay in bath for 15 to 20 minutes.
   - After the bath, remove the residue:
     —Scrub with a loofah sponge or washcloth and rinse the body well.
   - If skin irritation occurs, baths may need to be limited or avoided.
3. Taurine supplements
   Taurine, a sulfur amino acid, supports sulfation and detoxification. If your child has autism, only use taurine under the guidance of a health care practitioner. A subset of children with autism and a smaller subset with ADHD have metabolic disorders, some of which may render them intolerant to taurine. Starting with low doses will reveal any negative responses, which should resolve upon cessation. Blood and urine amino acid testing and a metabolic workup (to the degree determined necessary by a health care practitioner) will be helpful in guiding safe use of taurine.

TAURINE TOTAL DAILY GOAL DOSING

AGE	DOSE	FREQUENCY	TOTAL DAILY DOSE FROM ALL SOURCES
2 to 5	150 mg	1 or 2 times per day	300 mg
6 to 10	150 mg	2 times per day	300 mg
11 +	250 mg	2 times per day	500 mg

- Start at half of the lowest recommended dose and increase as tolerated.
- Watch for possible side effects and decrease the dose accordingly.
- If symptoms improve at lower than the goal dose, you may not need to continue to increase the dose.

Low Phenol/Low Salicylate Diet
If you have eliminated the artificial phenol/salicylate sources and the above measures are not sufficient, you may need to consider a trial elimination of all high-phenol foods. See section 6.2 Low Phenol/Salicylate (Feingold) Diet for information and resources for this diet.

Section E: High Glutamate and Need for GABA and Vitamin B$_6$

Glutamate is a transmitter with excitatory effects in the brain. Excitatory glutamate converts to the calming neurotransmitter, gamma-aminobutyric acid (GABA). Glutamate can increase in the brain if there is inefficiency in the glutamate decarboxylase enzyme or deficiency of vitamin B$_6$, which is necessary for the enzyme to function. The resulting symptoms include hyperactivity and also anxiety, tics, sleep problems, and irritability.

High glutamate is found in additives such as MSG and aspartame, which are the most problematic sources, and also in processed foods, milk products, grains, peanuts, and meats. The negative effects of glutamate in the brain are modulated by the calming amino acid and inhibitory neurotransmitter, GABA, which can be a helpful supplement for treating hyperactivity and also anxiety, OCD symptoms, language delay, perseverations, self-stimulatory behaviors, inattention, irritability, tics, and sleep problems.

What to Do and How to Do It
Provided here is a brief summary on GABA. For more information see section 4.11 GABA and Theanine.

GABA supplements
- GABA is best absorbed on an empty stomach, but may be taken with food.
- GABA's beneficial effects may affect dosing of medications used for ADHD, anxiety, and seizures.
- GABA should not be used if the child is already taking a medication that increases or potentially affects GABA, such as benzodiazepines, barbiturates, narcotics, and gabapentin.
- GABA, especially at higher doses, should only be used under the guidance of a health care practitioner.

GABA TOTAL DAILY GOAL DOSING

AGE	DOSE	FREQUENCY	TOTAL DAILY DOSE FROM ALL SOURCES
2 to 5	25 to 50 mg	2 times per day (breakfast and dinner)	50 to 100 mg
6 to 10	50 to 100 mg	2 times per day (breakfast and dinner)	100 to 200 mg
11 +	250 mg	1 or 2 times per day (breakfast and dinner)	250 to 500 mg

Side effects can include lethargy, excitability, and irritability.

Vitamin B₆

Vitamin B_6

Vitamin B_6 (pyridoxine) and its active form, pyridoxal-5′-phosphate (P5P), are necessary for the enzyme glutamate decarboxylase to convert excitatory glutamate to calming GABA.

What to Do and How to Do It

Some multiple vitamin supplements will have B_6 and/or P5P, which may be sufficient and not require additional supplementation. If they are not being used, supplementation may be necessary. For specifics on vitamin B_6 supplementation including products, see section 4.5 Methylation Nutrients.

Section F: Food Intolerances and Elimination of Opioid Food Culprits

Hyperactivity is a common effect of food intolerances. A full discussion of food intolerances is beyond the scope of this book. More information and resources are available in section 4.17 Digestive Enzymes and section 6.1 Gluten-Free Casein-Free Soy-Free (GFCFSF) Diet.

In short, food proteins, particularly those from milk (casein) and wheat (gluten), may be incompletely digested to peptides and enter the bloodstream from the intestine via an abnormally permeable intestinal lining (referred to as "leaky gut"). These partially digested protein peptides can potentially cross the blood–brain barrier, negatively affecting brain function, including contributing to hyperactivity, mood, attention, and behavior by several mechanisms:

- Blocking neurotransmitter messages
- Creating opiate-like doping effects from gluten (gliadorphin), milk casein (casomorphin), and soy
- Triggering brain inflammation

The most obvious symptom is a craving for the food opiate sources (gluten, milk products, and soy). In addition to hyperactivity and self-stimulatory behaviors, other symptoms include inattention, communication problems, poor eye contact, digestive problems, and irritability.

What to Do and How to Do It

Provided here is a brief summary of two main treatment strategies for food intolerances and the opiate-like peptide effect.

1. Gluten-Free Casein-Free Soy-Free (GFCFSF) Diet—Elimination Trial: the "gold standard" for treatment

- The most common problem food proteins are gluten, milk casein, and soy.
- Your child's body is the best test. Eliminate the food(s) to see whether behavior improves and reintroduce or challenge the body to see whether behavior worsens.
2. Digestive enzymes, including dipeptidyl peptidase-IV (DPP-IV)
   - More efficiently digest gluten, casein, soy, and other food proteins, carbohydrates, and fats.
   - Reduce the opioid load due to insufficient DPP-IV enzyme function; this can also "mimic" the diet.

Digestive Enzyme Supplements
See section 4.17 Digestive Enzymes for detailed information on specific enzyme products and dosing.

■ *2.11 Mood Issues*

Mood swings and difficulty regulating emotions can be seen in children with ADHD and autism. These symptoms may affect a child's self-esteem and social interactions. Depending on the degree of symptoms, the effect on a child's life may be profound.

Symptoms/signs your child may exhibit
- Significant changes in mood from day to day or within a day
- Unexplained irritability
- Sadness or depression

Main possible nutritional contributing factors
- Magnesium deficiency
- Food intolerances
- Intestinal yeast overgrowth
- Excess glutamate and need for GABA and low vitamin B_6
- Low serotonin
- Vitamin D deficiency
- Omega-3 DHA deficiency

DETERMINING WHICH SUPPLEMENTS AND DIET CHANGES MAY BE HELPFUL

IF YOUR CHILD HAS MOOD ISSUES AND SOME OF THE FOLLOWING SYMPTOMS	SEE THE APPLICABLE SECTION BELOW	DIETARY AND OTHER RECOMMENDATIONS	OTHER SOURCES OF INFORMATION
Constipation Sound sensitivity Easy startle Sleep disruption Excessive sighing	Section A: Magnesium	Higher intake of magnesium-rich foods: vegetables, beans, nuts, seeds, fruits	Chapter 4: section 4.8 Magnesium and Calcium

Mood Issues

Food cravings for milk casein and/or gluten and/or soy In a "fog" or "own world" Bowel problems Unexplained laughing High pain tolerance Poor eye contact Attention problems Language delays	Section B: Food Intolerances and Elimination of Opioid Food Culprits	Section B: Food Intolerances and Elimination of Opioid Food Culprits Gluten-Free Casein-Free Soy-Free (GFCFSF) diet	Chapter 4: section 4.17 Digestive Enzymes Chapter 6: section 6.1 GFCFSF Diet
Recurrent antibiotic use Thrush Diaper rashes Red ring around anus	Section C: Treatment of Intestinal Yeast Overgrowth	Section C: Treatment of Intestinal Yeast Overgrowth Anti-yeast diet	Chapter 4: section 4.16 Probiotics, section 4.6 Biotin, Chapter 6: section 6.4 Anti-Yeast Diet
Anxiety or OCD symptoms Sleep disruption Perseverations	Section E: Serotonin Support		
Scaly, cracked "ring around the mouth" Profuse sweating Delayed tooth eruption Bowing legs Bulging forehead "Knobby" knees or ankles Developmental delays	Section F: Vitamin D	Sun exposure, if tolerated	Chapter 4: section 4.2 Vitamin D
Cracking, peeling, chipping nails Language delays Vision dysfunction Excessive thirst Hard earwax	Section G: Essential Omega-3 Fatty Acids		Chapter 4: section 4.15 Essential Omega-3 Fatty Acids

Section A: Magnesium

Magnesium has overall calming effects on the nervous system. When magnesium is low, many behavioral effects can result, including mood dysregulation and irritability. Magnesium is a common nutritional deficiency in children with ADHD or autism. It is also a common deficiency in the general population.

What to Do and How to Do It

Provided here is a brief summary on magnesium. For thorough information and specific guidelines on dosing and side effects, see section 1.2 Magnesium.

Magnesium supplements
- Gentle (less laxative) stool effect: chelates, aspartates, glycinates, gluconates, and bisglycinates
- Laxative stool effect: citrates, chlorides, and sulfates

MAGNESIUM TOTAL DAILY GOAL DOSING

AGE	DOSE	FREQUENCY	TOTAL DAILY DOSE FROM ALL SOURCES
2 to 5	100 mg	1 or 2 times per day	200 mg
6 to 10	100 mg	2 or 3 times per day	300 mg
11 +	100 to 150 mg	2 or 3 times per day	450 mg

- Start at one-quarter to one-half of the recommended dose and increase the dose gradually every one to two days.
- Magnesium can cause loose stools or diarrhea.
- Watch for possible side effects and decrease the dose accordingly.
- If symptoms improve at lower than the goal dose, you may not need to continue to increase the dose.
- For higher-than-recommended doses, consult with a skilled health care practitioner.

Calcium

Calcium intake should be adequate when taking magnesium. Excess magnesium intake can lower calcium, and excess calcium intake can lower magnesium. It is important to have balance. If your child is not getting sufficient calcium from diet, a calcium supplement is indicated.

CALCIUM TOTAL DAILY GOAL DOSING

AGE	DOSE	FREQUENCY	TOTAL DAILY DOSE FROM ALL SOURCES
2 to 5	250 mg	2 times per day	500 mg
6 to 10	250 mg	3 times per day	750 mg
11 +	500 to 600 mg	2 times per day	1,000 to 1,200 mg

Section B: Food Intolerances and Elimination of Opioid Food Culprits

Mood and behavior issues can occur as a result of food intolerances. A full discussion of food intolerances is beyond the scope of this book. More information and resources are available in section 4.17 Digestive Enzymes and section 6.1 Gluten-Free Casein-Free Soy-Free (GFCFSF) Diet.

- The GFCF Diet Intervention—Autism Diet, www.gfcfdiet.com

In short, food proteins, particularly those from milk (casein) and wheat (gluten), may be incompletely digested to peptides and may enter the bloodstream from the intestine via an abnormally permeable intestinal lining (referred to as "leaky gut"). These partially digested protein peptides can potentially cross the blood–brain barrier, negatively affecting brain function, and issues contributing to hyperactivity, mood, attention, and behavior by several mechanisms:

- Blocking neurotransmitter messages
- Creating opiate-like doping effects from gluten (gliadorphin), milk casein (casomorphin), and soy
- Triggering brain inflammation

Mood Issues

The most obvious symptom is a craving for the food opiate sources (gluten, milk products, and soy). In addition to mood and behavior problems, other symptoms include hyperactivity, self-stimulatory behaviors, irritability, inattention, poor eye contact, and language delays. Effects may occur within an hour of consumption or be delayed up to seventy-two hours.

What to Do and How to Do It
Provided here is a brief summary of two main treatment strategies for food intolerances and the opiate-like peptide effect.
1. GFCFSF Diet—Elimination Trial: the "gold standard" for treatment
    • The most common problem food proteins are gluten, milk casein, and soy.
    • Your child's body is the best test. Eliminate the food(s) to see whether behavior improves and reintroduce or challenge the body to see whether behavior worsens.
2. Digestive enzymes, including dipeptidyl peptidase-IV (DPP-IV)
    • More efficiently digest gluten, casein, soy and other food proteins, carbohydrates, and fats.
    • Reduce the opioid load due to insufficient DPP-IV enzyme function; this can also "mimic" the diet.

Digestive Enzyme Supplements
See section 4.17 Digestive Enzymes for detailed information on specific enzyme products and dosing.

Section C: Treatment of Intestinal Yeast Overgrowth
Yeast organisms are normal residents of the intestinal tract. Contrary to popular understanding, problematic yeast overgrowth is common in children with a variety of digestive, behavioral, and developmental issues. Treatment may result in notable improvement in a subset of children.

Yeast overgrowth in the intestinal tract can result from inadequate beneficial bacteria because of antibiotic or steroid use, high sugar intake, and/or poor diet, including inadequate fiber. This can result in physical symptoms such as diaper rashes, oral thrush, skin conditions, intestinal inflammation, and abnormal stools. If yeast toxins are absorbed into the bloodstream through an abnormally permeable intestinal lining, behavioral symptoms can also result. These can include mood symptoms, inattention, anxiety, irritability, and silliness or unexplained laughing.

What to Do and How to Do It
Provided here is a brief summary on treatments for yeast overgrowth. For more thorough information, see section 2.18 Yeast Overgrowth, section 4.16 Probiotics, and section 4.6 Biotin.

Main beneficial treatments:
• Probiotics (beneficial bacteria)
• Biotin

- Antifungal (anti-yeast) medications or herbs
- Anti-yeast diet (anti-*Candida* diet)

Probiotics
Probiotics are beneficial live microorganisms called the microbiome, found throughout the body including the intestinal tract. There are more than 100 trillion good bacteria in the body with 500 to 1,000 different species (forty to fifty of which are main species) in the human gut. These beneficial bacteria serve many important functions, including maintaining healthy flora, preventing overgrowth of harmful pathogens and yeast, and producing healthy nutrients. For more detailed information on probiotics including specific products and dosing guidelines, see section 4.16 Probiotics.

Biotin
Biotin is a water-soluble B vitamin, manufactured in the human digestive tract by healthy flora. Antibiotics depress biotin production, which leads to yeast/fungal overgrowth. Biotin helps keep yeast in a less invasive form, which makes it easier to eradicate. Biotin is one of the safest supplements. It has no toxicity at any level. See section 4.6 The Helper B: Biotin for more information and dosing guidelines.

Antifungal Medications or Herbs
Probiotics help provide beneficial bacteria to the intestinal tract but do not directly kill yeast. Antifungal medications or herbs are used to kill yeast. Probiotics then help maintain good bacterial balance to prevent yeast overgrowth from recurring.

Antifungal treatments may include herbs or prescription medications. Depending on the amount of yeast present, intestinal symptoms and behavioral side effects from treatment may be significant. Known as "yeast die-off" symptoms, these may include irritability, behavioral regression, and flu-like symptoms. Because of the potential for significant side effects, antifungal treatment should be guided by a health care practitioner based on your child's history and, where possible, specific testing for yeast. See section 2.18 Yeast Overgrowth, for additional treatment information.

Anti-Yeast Diet
The anti-yeast diet avoids foods that "feed" yeast, such as sugars, yeast, starches, fruit juices, refined grains, and processed meats. Sugar is the primary culprit and should be limited or avoided. See section 6.4 Anti-Yeast Diet.

Section D: Excess Glutamate and Need for GABA and Vitamin B$_6$
Glutamate is a transmitter with excitatory effects in the brain. Excitatory glutamate converts to the calming neurotransmitter, gamma-aminobutyric acid (GABA). Glutamate can increase in the brain if there is inefficiency in the glutamate decarboxylase enzyme or deficiency of vitamin B$_6$, which is necessary for the enzyme to function.

Mood Issues

High glutamate is found in additives such as MSG and aspartame, which are the most problematic sources, and also in processed foods, milk products, grains, peanuts, and meats.

The negative effects of glutamate in the brain are modulated by the calming amino acid and inhibitory neurotransmitter GABA, which can be a helpful supplement for treating mood symptoms. It may also be helpful for anxiety, obsessive–compulsive symptoms, hyperactivity, language delay, perseverations, self-stimulatory behaviors, inattention, irritability, tics, and sleep problems.

What to Do and How to Do It

Provided here is a brief summary on GABA and B_6. For thorough information and specific guidelines on dosing and side effects, see section 4.11 GABA and Theanine, and section 4.5 Vitamin B_6.

- GABA is best absorbed on an empty stomach, but it may also be taken with food.
- GABA's beneficial effects may affect dosing of medications used for ADHD, anxiety, and seizures. Do not add GABA without discussing with your child's prescribing physician.
- GABA should not be used if the child is already taking a medication that increases or potentially affects GABA, such as benzodiazepines, barbiturates, narcotics, and gabapentin.
- GABA, especially at higher doses, should only be used under the guidance of a health care practitioner.
- Side effects can include lethargy, excitability, and irritability.

GABA TOTAL DAILY GOAL DOSING

AGE	DOSE	FREQUENCY	TOTAL DAILY DOSE FROM ALL SOURCES
2 to 5	25 to 50 mg	2 times per day (breakfast and dinner)	50 to 100 mg
6 to 10	50 to 100 mg	2 times per day (breakfast and dinner)	100 to 200 mg
11 +	250 mg	1 or 2 times per day (breakfast and dinner)	250 to 500 mg

Vitamin B_6

Vitamin B_6 (pyridoxine) and its active form, pyridoxal-5'-phosphate (P5P), are necessary for the enzyme glutamate decarboxylase to convert excitatory glutamate to calming GABA.

What to Do and How to Do It

Some multiple vitamin supplements will have B_6 and/or P5P, which may be sufficient and not require additional supplementation. If they are not being used, supplementation may be necessary. For specifics on B_6 supplementation including products, see section 4.5 Methylation Nutrients.

Section E: Serotonin Support

Serotonin is an important transmitter in the brain that affects mood, emotions, behavior, appetite, cognition, and attention. The amino acid tryptophan converts to 5-hydroxytryptophan (5-HTP), which then converts to serotonin; serotonin then converts to melatonin. Magnesium, vitamin B_3 (niacinamide), and vitamin B_6 (pyridoxine) are important in serotonin metabolism. Low levels of serotonin can result in depression, anxiety, obsessive–compulsive symptoms, self-stimulatory behaviors, repetitive movements, and sleep disorders.

What to Do and How to Do It

There are two main ways to raise serotonin:

1. Medications such as Selective Serotonin Reuptake Inhibitors (SSRIs):
   - SSRIs and 5-HTP raise serotonin levels in the brain but by different mechanisms.
   - Serotonin is released by neurons (nerve cells) in the brain and taken back up by these cells in order to be reused.
   - SSRIs block this uptake so that the serotonin effect is prolonged.
   - SSRIs must be prescribed and monitored by a physician.
2. Direct nutritional support of the serotonin pathway via tryptophan and 5-HTP
   - 5-HTP supplementation produces more serotonin directly as compared to L-tryptophan.
   - 5-HTP should be used only under the care of a health care practitioner.
   - The use of tryptophan and/or 5-HTP is not recommended when taking an SSRI medication because there is the risk for excessive serotonin.
   - Opposite reactions such as hyperactivity or insomnia, and/or manic symptoms may occur.
3. Serotonin nutrient cofactor supplementation:
   - Magnesium, zinc, iron, methylation support (B_6, B_{12}, and folinic acid), and vitamin B_3

These nutrients are essential to optimal serotonin metabolism. Use of a good multivitamin is a good start for providing these nutrient cofactors. More specific adjustment of cofactors is best done with guidance by a skilled health care practitioner (physician or nutritionist).

Section F: Vitamin D

Vitamin D deficiency is very common and can affect mood. Vitamin D deficiency can also affect development, attention, communication, immunity, and skin health. Risk factors for deficiency of vitamin D include inadequate sun exposure (or use of sunblock), darker skin pigmentation, obesity, breast feeding, low dietary intake, and fat malabsorption.

What to Do and How to Do It

Provided here is a brief summary on vitamin D. For more information on functions, products, dosing, and side effects, see section 4.2 Vitamin D.

Mood Issues

Vitamin D supplements
- Vitamin D_3 is available in capsules, tablets, and liquids.
- The micellized version of vitamin D_3 is a water-soluble form of vitamin D that is well absorbed and especially useful in malabsorption conditions.
- Vitamin D_3 (cholecalciferol) is the best form to use for supplementation.
- Vitamin D_2 (ergocalciferol) converts to vitamin D_3 and is less effective long term.
- The oil and micellized forms are preferred over the dry forms.

VITAMIN D TOTAL DAILY GOAL DOSING

AGE	DOSE	FREQUENCY
2 to 5	400 to 600 IU	Daily
6 to 10	600 to 800 IU	Daily
11 +	800 to 2,000 IU	Daily

- The total daily dose includes all sources such as D from cod liver oil and multiple vitamins.
- Do blood testing (25-hydroxy vitamin D) to guide dosing. The optimal goal level is 60 to 80 ng/mL.
- Adequate vitamin A intake must be maintained. See the vitamin A recommendations in section 4.1 Vitamin A.
- Higher doses may be required due to malabsorption or lab findings. This should be accomplished with a skilled health care practitioner.

Section G: Essential Omega-3 Fatty Acids

The essential omega-3 fatty acids are eicosapentaenoic acid (EPA) and docosahexaenoic acid (DHA). Almost 60 percent of the brain is composed of fat, with DHA being the primary structural component of the human brain and retina. DHA affects mood, behavior, cognition and attention.

What to Do and How to Do It

Provided here is a brief summary on omega-3 fatty acids. For thorough information and specific guidelines on supplement brands, dosing, and side effects, see section 4.15 Essential Omega-3 Fatty Acids.

The best food sources of omega-3 fatty acids are seafood. Those highest in mercury, PCBs, and other toxins include tomalley (crab mustard), farmed fish, trout, imported shrimp, and the large "steak" fish such as tuna, bluefish, swordfish, and shark. The safest choices include anchovies, sardines, domestic shrimp, rockfish, and tilapia.

Omega-3 supplements
- For mood and behavior and also communication, language, focus, and attention issues, we recommend that DHA amount be equal to or greater than the EPA.

- Use only direct-source EPA and DHA, which is more efficient than flax-seed-source ALA.
- Use toxin-free supplements: pharmaceutical grade or molecular distillation to remove toxins.

The following supplements have substantial levels of DHA:
- Barleans Omega Swirl
- Omega Cure (unflavored)
- Nordic Naturals ProOmega or Ultimate Omega
- Carlson Norwegian Cod Liver Oil with A and D$_3$
- Genestra Super DHA Liquid
- Nordic Naturals Baby's DHA (and EPA)
- Neuromins DHA caps (algae source DHA)
- Nordic Naturals ProDHA 1,000 soft gels

OMEGA-3 EPA AND DHA TOTAL DAILY GOAL DOSING

AGE	EPA	DHA	FREQUENCY
2 to 5	200 to 400 mg	200 to 400 mg	Daily with food
6 to 10	500 to 650 mg	400 to 500 mg	Daily with food
11 +	500 to 800 mg	500 to 650 mg	Daily with food

- Though DHA is preferred for assisting in mood, attention, focus, eye contact, and communication, EPA is also important and should be included.
- Higher than recommended doses of omega-3 fatty acids should only be given under the guidance of a skilled health care practitioner.

■ 2.12 *Pica*

Pica is the persistent ingestion of non-nutritive substances for a period of at least one month at an age at which this behavior is developmentally inappropriate (older than eighteen to twenty-four months). Children with pica have persistent and compulsive cravings to eat nonfood items. Depending on the severity, pica can lead to significant physical and mental symptoms.

There is debate over whether nutritional deficiencies cause pica or are the result of them. There are a few human and animal studies that associate pica with deficiencies (primarily iron, zinc, and calcium) that are responsive to supplementation. For example, beyond consuming nonfood substances, one of the hallmarks of iron deficiency is the craving for chewing ice, which ceases upon iron supplementation. The ingestion of nonfood substances, especially those that contain lead or other toxic metals, can decrease normal dietary intake of nutritive foods and/or also interfere with the absorption and utilization of necessary nutritional substances, especially zinc, iron, and calcium.

Pica is more common in those with developmental delays and autism and is not common in those with ADHD.

Symptoms/signs your child may exhibit

- Eating dirt, sand, chalk, paper, clay, paint, paint chips, hair, feces, or other nonfood items. (Note: Mouthing nonfood objects without consuming them is not considered pica.)
- Intestinal discomfort with possible intestinal blockage. This may occur if pica has been severe and results in an accumulated mass of ingested substances.
- Damaged teeth, depending on the substances consumed.
- Neurological symptoms including tremors.

Main possible contributing nutritional factors

- Zinc deficiency
- Iron deficiency
- Excess levels of lead and other toxic metals
- Excess copper levels

DETERMINING WHICH SUPPLEMENTS AND DIET CHANGES MAY BE HELPFUL

IF YOUR CHILD HAS PICA AND SOME OF THE FOLLOWING SYMPTOMS	SEE THE APPLICABLE SECTION BELOW	DIETARY AND OTHER RECOMMENDATIONS	OTHER SOURCES OF INFORMATION
Picky appetite White lines on nails Frequent illness Language delays Sensory sensitivities Growth delays Eczema, dermatitis Inattention Highly refined white diet Aversion to foods, especially vegetables	Section A: Zinc		Chapter 2: section 2.13 Picky Eating Chapter 4: section 4.9 Zinc
Fatigue and poor endurance Decreased energy Pale skin Pallor inside lower eyelid Nail-bed pallor upon pressure Dizzy upon standing Craving for chewing ice	Section B: Iron	Red meat, chicken, seafood, beans, nuts, seeds	
Anemia Neurological problems Reduced cognition	Section C: Testing for Lead and Other Toxic Metals		Chapter 5: section 5.1 Toxic Metals Chapter 3: section 3.2 Sulfation
Signs of zinc deficiency Symptoms of iron deficiency Anemia Hyperactivity Headaches Skin problems Depression	Section A: Zinc Section B: Iron Section D: Copper		Chapter 4: section 4.9 Zinc

Section A: Zinc

Zinc deficiency is extremely common in children with autism and is not unusual in children with ADHD. Zinc deficiency can occur if there is an intake of toxic metals. Zinc is necessary in the process of metabolizing and removing toxic metals. Toxic metals deplete zinc, and low zinc can result in the accumulation of toxic metals.

Metallothionein (MT) is a family of metal proteins that can provide protection against metal toxicity. MTs are dependent upon sufficient levels of zinc, copper, and selenium. Deficiencies in metallothionein function can result in toxic metal accumulation (especially cadmium, mercury, silver, and arsenic). Conversely, the accumulation of toxic metals can impair metallothionein function. Zinc is also depleted by a high carbohydrate/glycemic diet, medications such as antacids, and innately higher metabolic needs.

What to Do and How to Do It
Provided here is a brief summary on zinc. For thorough information and specific guidelines on dosing and side effects see section 4.9 Zinc.

Zinc supplements
- Well tolerated: gluconates, chelates, citrates, acetates, picolinates, chlorides, and bisglycinates
- Strong taste, needs disguising: sulfates

ZINC TOTAL DAILY GOAL DOSING

AGE	DOSE	FREQUENCY	TOTAL DAILY DOSE FROM ALL SOURCES
2 to 5	5 to 10 mg	1 or 2 times per day	10 to 20 mg
6 to 10	10 mg	2 times per day	20 mg
11 +	10 to 15 mg	2 times per day	20 to 30 mg

For optimal oral absorption, an empty stomach is best, but it may not be feasible if nausea occurs. Large doses can cause gastric discomfort, nausea, and inhibit the digestive enzyme DPP-IV (digests opioids from gluten and casein). In addition:
- Avoid or limit giving zinc at the same time as interfering nutrients: calcium, iron, folate, and phosphorylated nutrients (R5P, P5P, phosphatidylcholine), though this may not always be feasible.
- Zinc excess can lower copper levels. Copper levels need to be maintained.
- If copper levels are elevated, zinc supplementation is helpful in normalizing copper levels.
- Higher doses may be required because of poor absorption, antacid use, the load of toxic metals, and/or specific lab findings. This should be accomplished with a skilled health care practitioner.

Pica

Zinc Testing

Your child's physician can order blood testing for zinc deficiency. For zinc testing we recommend red-blood-cell zinc testing, as this is a much more sensitive measure than the more commonly ordered serum zinc test.

The Zinc Tally Taste Test (a zinc sulfate solution) is a screening test for zinc deficiency. When zinc levels are poor, the solution tastes like water. When zinc levels are good, the taste is strong, even offensive. See page 213.

Section B: Iron

Iron-deficiency anemia is commonly associated with pica and also with accumulation of toxic metals such as lead, copper, mercury, and others.

Body stores of iron as shown by low ferritin levels on blood testing decline first, prior to serum iron declining. These deficits occur before the complete blood count indicates anemia. For this reason, symptoms such as inattention, poor endurance, lethargy, or fatigue may show up before the complete blood count (CBC) reveals there is a problem.

What to Do and How to Do It

Provided here is a brief summary on iron. For thorough information and specific guidelines on dosing and side effects, see the section on iron in chapter 4.

Iron should never be given without blood testing to document whether your child has a need for it. If levels of iron are too high or there is a metabolic disorder in which iron accumulates in the tissues, iron supplementation can be damaging and even toxic. Consider these tests to determine levels: CBC, serum iron, TIBC, percent saturation, and serum ferritin (a measure of iron stores). When taking iron, routine follow-up blood testing is critical.

Iron dietary sources
- The richest and best-absorbed iron (heme) is found in meats, especially liver.
- Plant sources of iron (nonheme) are less well absorbed (beans, nuts, seeds, and spinach).

Iron supplements:
- All forms of iron supplements can darken the stool (depending upon the dose).
- Iron supplements can cause constipation, especially the sulfate forms.
- Forms that are well tolerated by the digestive tract are ferrous fumarate, gluconate, chelates, and bisglycinate.

IRON TOTAL DAILY GOAL DOSING

AGE	DOSE	FREQUENCY	TOTAL DAILY DOSE FROM ALL SOURCES
2 to 5	7 to 10 mg	Daily	7 to 10 mg
6 to 10	10 mg	Daily	10 mg
11 +	8 to 10 mg	Daily	8 to 10 mg

- We strongly recommend that you do not give iron to treat pica without consulting a physician and having appropriate blood testing. Doses based on blood testing may be higher than those listed in the above table.
- Iron is best taken at a different time from calcium, zinc, phosphorus, fiber, and vitamin E.
- For better absorption, iron is best taken with vitamin C.
- The main side effect of treatment with iron is constipation, which can be resolved by adding magnesium and/or vitamin C. See section 2.6 Constipation.

Section C: Testing for Lead and Other Toxic Metals

In pica, suspect elevated lead if there is consumption of lead paint chips, dirt, stones, and other contaminated materials. Other sources of lead can include contaminated food, contaminated water supply, and industrial exposure. Elevated lead can cause numerous medical problems ranging from constipation to neurological problems, depending on the degree of elevation. Blood lead testing can be ordered by your child's physician.

Testing for other toxic metals, including mercury, requires sophisticated assessments and is beyond the scope of this book. As stated before, low ferritin can indicate a burden of one or more toxic metals. We have found that hair analysis is a reasonable screening tool for identifying recent exposure to or elimination of toxic metals. Hair analysis is a permanent chronological record of what is moving in and out of the body. Hair measures what has been present in the blood in the preceding six to eight weeks. Blood testing is generally not helpful, because metals either deposit in other tissues or are excreted from the body and are not typically found in blood unless there is recent or ongoing significant exposure.

All people are exposed to toxic metals in the environment. The difference is based upon how each individual metabolically handles the toxins. Those with impaired metabolic processes such as in methylation (dependent upon B vitamins) and sulfation (dependent upon cysteine, N-acetyl cysteine, alpha-lipoic acid, and glutathione) have an inability to metabolize and rid toxins efficiently. When toxic metals are present, important vitamins, minerals, and amino acids decline and, conversely, when vitamins, minerals, and amino acids are deficient, toxic metals are more likely to accumulate.

Treatment for metal toxicity is beyond the scope of this book. The nutritional focus for preventing toxic metal accumulation involves identifying and treating the nutritional deficiencies and poorly functioning metabolic pathways that can lead to toxic metal accumulation.

For more information on lead and other toxic metals, see section 5.1 Toxic Metals.

Section D: Copper

Copper is an essential trace element critical in numerous metabolic processes including hemoglobin metabolism. Insufficient copper can cause an anemia that is nonresponsive to iron supplementation. Conversely, elevated copper can suppress iron, leading to anemia as well. Copper and zinc are also interrelated in that high copper intake can lower zinc levels and high zinc intake can lower copper levels.

Elevated copper is of significant concern because it can lead to toxicity and elicit symptoms ranging from headaches and hyperactivity to liver and kidney damage. There are genetic conditions in which copper accumulates abnormally, requiring medical treatment.

Diet and supplements rarely cause toxic levels of copper, but they can exacerbate high copper levels; hence medical supervision and assessment are needed prior to supplementation. The most common sources of non-nutritive copper responsible for most of the elevated or toxic levels include contaminated water, unlined copper cookware, and industrial exposures.

Elevated copper can be seen in both autism and ADHD. Testing and treatment for copper should be accomplished by a health care practitioner. Tests to consider include serum copper, red-blood-cell copper, and serum ceruloplasmin. It is especially important to test for copper if your child is on higher doses of zinc (e.g., 40 mg/day or higher) as copper deficiency is not uncommon when this is the case.

■ 2.13 Picky Eating

Picky eating is extremely common in children with autism, who may exhibit very restricted food choices. When underlying factors are addressed, food selection may gradually broaden, resulting in a healthier diet.

Symptoms/signs your child may exhibit
- Overall limited food choices
- Unusual food preferences
- Varied appetite for baby food, which declines after introduction of solid table foods
- Preference for the "white" diet (bread, pasta, cheese, milk products, sweets)
- Preference for very spicy or strong tasting food
- Strong aversion to vegetables
- Aversion to certain food textures, colors, smells, or temperatures

Main possible contributing nutritional factors
- Zinc deficiency
- Oral-motor tone issues and sensory sensitivities
- Opiate peptide issues
- Presence of toxic metals (e.g., lead, mercury, and others)

DETERMINING WHICH SUPPLEMENTS AND DIET CHANGES MAY BE HELPFUL

IF YOUR CHILD HAS A PICKY APPETITE AND SOME OF THE FOLLOWING SYMPTOMS	SEE THE APPLICABLE SECTION BELOW	DIETARY AND OTHER RECOMMENDATIONS	OTHER SOURCES OF INFORMATION
White lines on nails Frequent illness Eczema/dermatitis Elevated toxic metals Language delays Developmental delays Growth delays Sensory sensitivities Inattention Highly refined white diet Aversion to foods, especially vegetables	Section A: Zinc		Chapter 4: section 4.9 Zinc
Food cravings for milk casein and/or gluten and/or soy In a "fog" or "own world" Bowel problems Unexplained laughing High pain tolerance Poor eye contact Mood problems Language delays Attention issues Cognitive problems	Section B: Food Intolerances and Elimination of Opioid Food Culprits	Section B: Food Intolerances and Elimination of Opioid Food Culprits Gluten-Free Casein-Free Soy-Free (GFCFSF) diet	Chapter 4: section 4.17 Digestive Enzymes Chapert 6: Section 6.1 GFCFSF diet
Oral-motor tone issues Sensory sensitivities Speech delays	Section C: Strategies for Oral-Motor Tone Issues and Sensory Sensitivities Section A: Zinc		"Trojan Horse Technique" in *The Kid-Friendly ADHD & Autism Cookbook* by the authors
Eating nonfood items Neurological symptoms, including tremors			Chapter 2: section 2.12 Pica

Picky Eating

Section A: Zinc

Zinc is critical in sensory development and function. Zinc deficiency can cause a loss of taste directly at the level of the taste buds (on the tongue, palate, and throat) and also affects perception of taste in the brain. Once taste is diminished, altered, or lost, many foods can become unpalatable and even offensive. As zinc status declines, taste perception decreases and aversions increase, especially to vegetables and often to specific textures, colors, and smells. Some children will even gag at the sight of a food that is offensive.

Perception is reality and the child is responding reasonably to the taste perceived. The child then limits choices to a few foods such as sweets, pasta, breads, cold cereals, macaroni and cheese, and ice cream. Some even prefer stronger tasting or spicier foods in an attempt to detect enough taste to make the food tolerable. Other children will simply avoid the unpalatable foods.

Zinc deficiency or functional deficit is a common finding in autism and not unusual in children with ADHD. It also affects development, attention, communication, immunity, glucose control, and vitamin A transport.

What to Do and How to Do It
Provided here is a brief summary on zinc. For thorough information and specific guidelines on dosing and side effects, see section 4.9 Zinc.

Zinc supplements
• Well tolerated: gluconates, chelates, citrates, acetates, picolinates, chlorides, and bisglycinates
• Strong taste, needs disguising: sulfates

ZINC TOTAL DAILY GOAL DOSING

AGE	DOSE	FREQUENCY	TOTAL DAILY DOSE FROM ALL SOURCES
2 to 5	5 to 10 mg	1 or 2 times per day	10 to 20 mg
6 to 10	10 mg	2 times per day	20 mg
11 +	10 to 15 mg	2 times per day	20 to 30 mg

For optimal oral absorption, an empty stomach is best, but it may not be feasible if nausea occurs. Large doses can cause gastric discomfort, nausea, and inhibit the digestive enzyme DPP-IV (digests opioids from gluten and casein). In addition:
• Avoid or limit giving zinc at the same time as interfering nutrients: calcium, iron, folate, and phosphorylated nutrients (R5P, P5P, phosphatidylcholine); this may not always be feasible.
• Zinc excess can lower copper levels. Copper levels need to be maintained.
• Use the Zinc Tally Taste Test on page 213 for evaluating progress with zinc supplementation.
• Higher doses may be required because of malabsorption, antacid use, the presence of toxic metals, or lab findings. Higher dosing should be accomplished with a health care practitioner.

Section B: Food Intolerances and Elimination of Opioid Food Culprits
Picky appetite is often noted in food intolerances. A full discussion of food intolerances is beyond the scope of this book. More information and resources are available in section 4.17 Digestive Enzymes and section 6.1 Gluten-Free Casein-Free Soy-Free (GFCFSF) Diet.

In short, food proteins, particularly those from milk (casein) and wheat (gluten), may be incompletely digested to peptides and may enter the bloodstream from the intestine via an abnormally permeable intestinal lining (referred to as "leaky gut"). These partially digested protein peptides can potentially cross the blood–brain barrier, negatively affecting brain function by several mechanisms, such as:
• Blocking neurotransmitter messages

- Creating opiate-like doping effects from gluten (gliadorphin), milk casein (casomorphin), and soy
- Triggering brain inflammation

Children who have high levels of opiate-like peptides may crave these opiate-creating foods so strongly that they are not interested in other foods. This can contribute to picky eating. Consider this if your child has strong cravings for food opiate sources (gluten, milk products, and soy). Other symptoms can include inattention, language delays, poor eye contact, hyperactivity, irritability, and increased self-stimulation and repetitive actions. Effects may occur within an hour of consumption or be delayed up to seventy-two hours.

What to Do and How to Do It
Provided here is a brief summary of two main treatment strategies food intolerances and the opioid effect.
1. GFCFSF Diet—Elimination Trial: the "gold standard" for treatment
   - The most common problem food proteins are gluten, milk casein, and soy.
   - Your child's body is the best test. Eliminate the food(s) to see whether behavior improves and reintroduce or challenge the body to see whether behavior worsens.
2. Digestive enzymes, including dipeptidyl peptidase-IV (DPP-IV)
   - More efficiently digest gluten, casein, soy and other food proteins, carbohydrates, and fats.
   - Reduce the opioid load due to insufficient DPP-IV enzyme function; this can also "mimic" the diet.

Digestive Enzyme Supplements
See section 4.17 Digestive Enzymes for detailed information on specific enzyme products and dosing.

Section C: Strategies for Oral-Motor Tone Issues and Sensory Sensitivities
Beyond the issues with taste, many children with autism and some children with ADHD also have issues with processing sensory information including sounds, touch, movement, smells, and food textures. Zinc is critical to sensory development affecting not just food taste, appearance, and smell perception, but how textures are perceived and tolerated.

Poor oral muscle tone can be present when there are problems with food textures. Muscle tone depends upon adequate zinc (and B_6) for amino acid utilization by tissues. Poor muscle tone of mouth muscles can also affect speech. The child will find it difficult to eat solid, textured foods and will prefer pureed, soft, "baby" foods.

When oral-motor development is delayed, the ability to handle solid foods and textures declines. The combination of food tasting unpleasant along with the offensive texture results in the food becoming an aversion.

Once a child has a bad experience with a food, it can be very difficult to get the child to try that food again. Food reactions are visceral experiences. For

Picky Eating

example, if you have ever had the coincidental misfortune of having a stomach virus occur around the time you ate a particular food, those two experiences are then linked in a powerful way. The aversion can continue for quite some time and be difficult to overcome. It is an innate reaction and not a logical response. We are hardwired to reject any food perceived as harmful. A child who does not possess the cognitive abilities to override the innate connection may take a long time before being willing to try that specific food again.

What to Do and How to Do It

Zinc is a critical nutrient in amino acid metabolism that affects muscle tone. See section A for supplementation information.

Vitamin B_6 (pyridoxine) and its active form, pyridoxal-5'-phosphate (P5P), are necessary in amino acid metabolism. Some multiple vitamin supplements will have B_6 and/or P5P, which may be sufficient and additional supplementation may not be required. If they are not being used, supplementation may be necessary.

VITAMIN B_6 TOTAL DAILY GOAL DOSING

FORM OF B_6	AGE	DAILY DOSE WITH FOOD BEFORE NOON	TOTAL DAILY DOSE FROM ALL SOURCES
Vitamin B_6 (pyridoxine)	2 to 5	10 to 15 mg	30 mg
	6 to 10	20 to 30 mg	60 mg
	11 +	50 mg	100 mg
P5P (pyridoxal-5'-phosphate)	2 to 5	5 mg	5 mg
	6 to 10	10 mg	10 mg
	11 +	15 mg	15 mg

- B_6 is more effective if taken with magnesium.
- If sulfate is low, avoid the P5P form of vitamin B_6.
- Therapeutic doses beyond recommendations must be accomplished under the guidance of a health care practitioner.

Feeding Strategies and Therapies

Often when zinc deficiency is treated, children are willing to expand their diets and retry old foods or try new foods as they discover the good taste. However, even when zinc and B_6 deficiencies are treated and taste and oral tone improve, some children with sensory sensitivities may continue to refuse foods because of past negative associations. The following should help:

- Feed according to the child's sensory developmental level, not his or her chronological age.
- Children with oral-motor tone problems find it difficult to manipulate more solid foods and increase rejection or aversion to specific foods. In fact, many parents will state the following: "He ate so well when he was on baby food and when solid foods were introduced, he refused to eat most of them." It is not a problem to go back to the "baby food" style purees that

are easy for the child to use. As nutrition and feeding therapies work together, the child will be able to expand to foods with more textures.

The Trojan Horse Technique

To get your child acclimated to new foods, the Trojan Horse Technique is most helpful. This involves disguising and hiding the new food in with a food the child already likes and eats. Mix the well-liked food with the new food. Puree them together thoroughly so that there are no "lumps or bumps" and that it is homogenous in texture and color. In a larger portion of the well-liked food, hand-mix the puree, starting with small amounts.

Hide the purees in fruit smoothies, meatballs, soups, spaghetti sauce, pizza sauce (under the cheese), healthy muffins and cookies, and even in macaroni and cheese sauce (regular or gluten-free casein-free versions). Spaghetti sauce can become vegetable and meat spaghetti sauce.

Many of our families have developed what we call "muffin casseroles," which can include fruits, beans, vegetables, and meats. Making these "casseroles" usually begins by adding pureed fruit to the batter, then gradually expanding.

Consider adding a vegetable juice to the child's favorite fruit juice. Both should be natural juices that can be diluted with water. However, some children have extremely narrow choices and you may have to start with whatever juice the child is consuming. Try carrot juice with orange juice, then add another vegetable juice and expand as tolerance improves. Opaque sippy cups can hide the color changes that may occur. There are fruit and vegetable "green" powders available that can be added to any of the foods suggested.

If more protein is needed, there are many clever ways to increase it. If eggs are tolerated, add more eggs, especially the protein-high whites. (Do not add raw eggs to smoothies; avidin in the egg destroys biotin.) This works for batters, breads, and meatballs. Rice, whey, pea protein powders, and nut flours can also be added to batters, breads, and smoothies made with milk or milk substitutes (coconut, nut, rice, hemp). Taste and texture determine acceptance.

This technique helps the child adjust subtly to a new taste, eventually becoming more ready to accept the foods in their more visible form. The combining of the new food with the well-liked food increases the acceptance because the child's sensory system links the previously "yucky" taste with the good taste. This accomplishes two important goals: improving the child's intake of important nutritional foods and expanding his or her food choices.

Use the EAT Strategy to Introduce New Foods

For an interesting, easy-to-follow book on dealing with feeding issues, read *What's Eating Your Child* by Kelly Dorfman, M.S., L.D.N. (www.kellydorfman.com). Dorfman outlines the EAT technique, which stands for:

Eliminate any reactive or unhealthy food from the diet

Add one new food, especially one that is similar to a food already enjoyed

Try one bite of the same new food daily for weeks

Picky Eating

Feeding Specialists

If you have supplemented appropriately, incorporated the Trojan Horse Technique and the additional feeding advice, and the problem continues, consider a feeding specialist who understands sensory issues.

Many children are experiencing a form of post-traumatic stress disorder based on the way the child experienced food taste, texture, color, and smell. The deficiencies and oral-motor tone issues lead to the unpleasant perceptions that are the child's reality. This information becomes hardwired and is difficult to change, but it can be accomplished with diligence and expert help.

Melissa Olive, Ph.D., B.C.B.A.-D., certified in behavioral analysis and expert in feeding problems, and Kelly Barnhill, C.N., C.C.N., a nutritionist with expertise in feeding problems, describe the following helpful strategies:

The most successful programs try to expand food acceptance through behavior modification involving coming to the table, sitting at the table, accepting new foods, and eventually self-feeding. This involves reinforcing the targeted behavior with appropriate rewards that are highly preferred by the child (toys, books, a favorite healthy food, video, TV). The keys are taking baby steps, moving steadily slowly, and using small amounts of foods.

For some children, food may be placed in the room where it can be seen, then ultimately closer to the child, followed by touching the food with the fingers. Then, children are introduced one new food, one bite at a time, in the following sequential manner:

- Touch lip
- Touch tongue
- Enter mouth and spit
- Chew and spit
- Chew and swallow

After the child is able to chew and swallow each food without complaint, then the bites are increased sequentially. Consistency is important in achieving success. These types of feeding interventions are best guided by a therapist.

■ 2.14 *Sensory Sensitivities*

Difficulties with processing and regulation of sensory input are extremely common in both children with autism and ADHD. Depending on the degree of symptoms, sensory issues can result in significant limitations to a child's ability to comfortably exist in his or her environment and to be available for appropriate social interaction. The discomfort from poor sensory processing can also result in irritability, anxiety, and mood issues.

Symptoms/signs your child may exhibit

- Sensitivity to sounds (e.g., vacuum cleaner, hair dryer, flushing toilets, general loud environments)
- Sensitivity to touch (e.g., tags on clothing, light touch, tickling)

- Sensitivity to smells or light
- Need for proprioceptive (pressure) input (e.g., seeks out bear hugs, crawls under sofa cushions or into tight spaces)
- Need for vestibular input (e.g., likes to be upside down, craves swinging)
- Need for movement, fidgeting, climbing, "hyperactivity"
- Aversion to food textures, appearance, smell, temperature, and/or taste

Main possible contributing factors
- Magnesium deficiency
- Zinc deficiency
- Food sensitivities (e.g., to gluten, casein, and/or soy)

DETERMINING WHICH SUPPLEMENTS AND DIET CHANGES MAY BE HELPFUL

IF YOUR CHILD HAS SENSORY SENSITIVITIES AND SOME OF THE SYMPTOMS BELOW	SEE THE APPLICABLE SECTION BELOW	DIETARY AND OTHER RECOMMENDATIONS	OTHER SOURCES FOR INFORMATION
Constipation Sound sensitivity Easy startle Sleep disruption Mood issues Excessive sighing Hyperactivity	Section A: Magnesium	Higher intake of magnesium-rich foods: vegetables, beans, nuts, seeds, fruits	Chapter 4: section 4.8 Magnesium and Calcium
Picky appetite White lines on nails Frequent illness Eczema/dermatitis Elevated toxic metals Language delays Developmental delays Growth delays Inattention Highly refined "white" diet	Section B: Zinc		Chapter 4: section 4.9 Zinc
Food cravings for milk casein and/or gluten and/or soy In a "fog" or "own world" Bowel problems Unexplained laughing High pain tolerance Poor eye contact Mood problems Attention problems Language delays	Section C: Food Intolerances and Elimination of Opioid Food Culprits	Section C: Food Intolerances and Elimination of Opioid Food Culprits Gluten-Free Casein-Free Soy-Free (GFCFSF) diet	Chapter 4: section 4.17 Digestive Enzymes Chapter 6: section 6.1 GFCFSF Diet

Section A: Magnesium

Magnesium has calming effects on the nervous system. Low magnesium levels result in neuromuscular excitability, eliciting an exaggerated response to the environment, including easy startle, anxiety, and exaggerated reactions to clothing, sound, light, and pressure. Some children will be unusually emotionally sensitive. Additional deficiency symptoms include sensory-seeking behaviors,

Sensory Sensitivities

obsessive–compulsive symptoms, rigidity, constipation, muscle spasms, repetitive behavior, and fidgeting or hyperactivity. Magnesium is a common nutritional deficiency in children with ADHD and autism, as well as in the general population.

What to Do and How to Do It
Provided here is a brief summary on magnesium. For thorough information, see section 4.8 Magnesium and Calcium.

Magnesium supplements
• Gentle (less laxative) stool effect: chelates, aspartates, glycinates, gluconates, and bisglycinates
• Laxative stool effect: citrates, chlorides, sulfates

MAGNESIUM TOTAL DAILY GOAL DOSING

AGE	DOSE	FREQUENCY	TOTAL DAILY DOSE FROM ALL SOURCES
2 to 5	100 mg	1 or 2 times per day	200 mg
6 to 10	100 mg	2 or 3 times per day	300 mg
11 +	100 to 150 mg	2 or 3 times per day	450 mg

• Start at one-quarter to one-half of the recommended dose and increase the dose gradually every one to two days.
• Magnesium can cause loose stools or diarrhea, which then can deplete magnesium levels.
• Watch for possible side effects and decrease the dose accordingly.
• If symptoms improve at lower than the goal dose, you may not need to continue to increase the dose.
• For higher-than-recommended doses, consult with a health care practitioner.

Calcium
Calcium intake should be adequate when taking magnesium. Excess magnesium intake can lower calcium, and excess calcium intake can lower magnesium. It is important to have balance. If your child is not getting sufficient calcium from diet, a calcium supplement is indicated.

CALCIUM TOTAL DAILY GOAL DOSING

AGE	DOSE	FREQUENCY	TOTAL DAILY DOSE FROM ALL SOURCES
2 to 5	250 mg	2 times per day	500 mg
6 to 10	250 mg	3 times per day	750 mg
11 +	500 to 600 mg	2 times per day	1,000 to 1,200 mg

Section B: Zinc
Zinc deficiency is extremely common in children with autism and is not unusual

in children with ADHD. It affects brain pruning (the normal process of regulating the number of neurons and synapses in the brain to allow it to function more efficiently) and sensory development and function. Symptoms may include the full range between sensory seeking and sensory avoidant behaviors. The sensory systems affected are touch, taste, smell, eye contact, vision processing, auditory processing, and texture perception. The perception is reality; therefore, the child's response to sensory stimuli is a reasonable response to the way they are perceived. Additional symptoms include poor attention, developmental delays, communication delays, vitamin A deficiency, immune dysfunction, and poor glucose control.

What to Do and How to Do It
Provided here is a brief summary on zinc. For thorough information and specific guidelines on dosing and side effects, see section 4.9 Zinc.
  Zinc supplements
• Well tolerated: gluconates, chelates, citrates, acetates, picolinates, chlorides, and bisglycinates
• Strong taste, needs disguising: sulfates

ZINC TOTAL DAILY GOAL DOSING

AGE	DOSE	FREQUENCY	TOTAL DAILY DOSE FROM ALL SOURCES
2 to 5	5 to 10 mg	1 or 2 times per day	10 to 20 mg
6 to 10	10 mg	2 times per day	20 mg
11 +	10 to 15 mg	2 times per day	20 to 30 mg

For optimal oral absorption, an empty stomach is best, but it may not be feasible if nausea occurs. Large doses can cause gastric discomfort, nausea, and inhibit the digestive enzyme DPP-IV (digests opioids from gluten and casein). In addition:
• Avoid or limit giving zinc at the same time as interfering nutrients such as calcium, iron, folate, and phosphorylated nutrients (R5P, P5P, phosphatidylcholine); this may not always be feasible.
• Zinc excess can lower copper levels. Copper levels need to be maintained.
• Use the Zinc Tally Taste Test in section 4.9 for evaluating progress with zinc supplementation.
• Higher doses may be required due to poor absorption, antacid use, the presence of toxic metals, or lab findings of deficiency. This should be accomplished with a health care practitioner.

Section C: Food Intolerances and Elimination of Opioid Food Culprits
Food intolerances impact significantly on sensory sensitivities. A full discussion of food intolerances is beyond the scope of this book. More information and resources are available in section 4.17 Digestive Enzymes and section 6.1 Gluten-Free Casein-Free Soy-Free (GFCFSF) Diet.

In short, food proteins, particularly those from milk (casein) and wheat (gluten), may be incompletely digested to peptides and may enter the blood-stream from the intestine via an abnormally permeable intestinal lining (referred to as "leaky gut"). These partially digested protein peptides can potentially cross the blood–brain barrier, negatively affecting brain function, and contributing to mood, attention, and behavior by several mechanisms:
- Blocking neurotransmitter messages
- Creating opiate-like doping effects from gluten (gliadorphin), milk casein (casomorphin), and soy
- Triggering brain inflammation

The most obvious symptom is craving for the food opiate sources (gluten, milk products, and soy). The opioid effect can also contribute to inattention, language and communication delays, poor eye contact, irritability, and increased self-stimulating behavior. Effects may occur within an hour of consumption or be delayed up to seventy-two hours.

What to Do and How to Do It
Provided here is a brief summary of two main treatment strategies for food intolerances and the opioid effect.
1. GFCFSF Diet—Elimination Trial: the "gold standard" for treatment
   - The most common problem food proteins are gluten, milk casein, and soy.
   - Your child's body is the best test. Eliminate the food(s) to see whether behavior improves and reintroduce or challenge the body to see whether behavior worsens.
2. Digestive enzymes, including dipeptidyl peptidase-IV (DPP-IV)
   - More efficiently digest gluten, casein, soy and other food proteins, carbohydrates, and fats.
   - Reduce the opioid load due to insufficient DPP-IV enzyme function; this can also "mimic" the diet.

Digestive Enzyme Supplements
See section 4.17 Digestive Enzymes for detailed information on specific enzyme products and dosing.

■ 2.15 *Silly Behavior and Inappropriate Giggling/Laughing*
It is not uncommon for children with autism to have episodes of unexplained giggling or laughing. This can happen at any time during the day and may also occur as part of night waking.

Symptoms/signs your child may exhibit
- Laughing or giggling without obvious reason
- Waking at night and laughing

Main possible contributing nutritional factors
- Phenol sensitivity
- Opiate-like peptides from casein, gluten, or soy
- Intestinal yeast overgrowth

DETERMINING WHICH SUPPLEMENTS AND DIET CHANGES MAY BE HELPFUL

IF YOUR CHILD HAS UNEXPLAINED GIGGLING/ LAUGHING AND SOME OF THE FOLLOWING SYMPTOMS	SEE THE APPLICABLE SECTION BELOW	DIETARY AND OTHER RECOMMENDATIONS	OTHER SOURCES OF INFORMATION
Red cheeks or ears without obvious explanation Sweating at night Hyperactivity Difficulty sleeping	Section A: Phenol Sensitivity	Low phenol diet Avoidance of salicylate medications and artificial additives, coloring, flavoring	Chapter 6: section 6.2 Low Phenol Diet
Food cravings for milk casein and/or gluten and/or soy In a "fog" or "own world" Bowel problems High pain tolerance Poor eye contact Mood problems Attention problems Language delays	Section B: Food Intolerances and Elimination of Opioid Food Culprits	Section B: Food Intolerances and Elimination of Opioid Food Culprits Elimination of the opioid food culprits: gluten, milk products, soy Gluten-Free Casein-Free Soy-Free (GFCFSF) diet	Chapter 4: section 4.17 Digestive Enzymes Chapter 6: section 6.1 GFCFSF diet
Recurrent antibiotic use Coated tongue Thrush Diaper rashes Red ring around anus	Section C: Treatment of Intestinal Yeast Overgrowth	Section C: Treatment of Intestinal Yeast Overgrowth Anti-yeast diet	Chapter 2: section 2.18 Yeast Overgrowth Chapter 4: section 4.16 Probiotics, section 4.6 Biotin Chapter 6: section 6.4 Anti-Yeast Diet

Silly Behavior

Section A: Phenol Sensitivity

Phenols are naturally occurring beneficial nutritional chemicals found in high concentration in a variety of foods, especially cow's milk products, apples, bananas, red grapes, berries, and tomatoes. The enzyme, phenol sulfotransferase (PST), uses sulfate to metabolize phenols. When PST and/or sulfate is deficient, phenols fail to be metabolized well and sensitivity occurs. For a subset of children, especially those with autism, sulfate levels are inadequate.

- Aspirin and artificial food additives, coloring, and flavorings are the most significant load on the PST system.
- Excess B_6 as pyridoxal-5'-phosphate can inhibit the enzyme and make it worse.
- Symptoms of phenol sensitivity include hyperactivity, red cheeks or red ears without an obvious explanation, night sweating, poor sleep, and/or unexplained giggling or silliness.

What to Do and How to Do It

There are three treatment options for phenol sensitivity:

- Provision of sulfate to help the PST enzyme work better
- Removal of items with the highest phenol content: medications and all synthetic additives in the diet.
- Limiting of foods with high phenol content

How to Provide Sulfate

Sulfate improves PST enzyme function and enhances detoxification. The following three strategies should be helpful:

1. Magnesium sulfate topical lotion
   - Magnesium sulfate lotion 100 mg dose per gram of cream (made by Kirkman Labs)
   - Apply lotion to muscle areas where absorption is the highest: shoulders, back, or calves. Use the chart below for dosing recommendations.
   - Massage in thoroughly. It may take 30 minutes to absorb, after which other lotions can be applied.
   - Rotate the application sites to reduce skin irritation.
   - If skin irritation or rash occurs, consider a custom compounded hypoallergenic lotion.
   - Topical magnesium sulfate lotion is not a good source of magnesium.

MAGNESIUM SULFATE TOPICAL LOTION TOTAL DAILY GOAL DOSING

Starting dose	100 mg in the morning
After 2 to 3 days	100 mg morning and evening
After 2 to 3 more days	100 mg morning, noon (or after school), and evening

2. Epsom salts and baking soda baths
   - To a bath of tolerated hot water add 1 to 2 cups Epsom salts and 1 to 2 cups bicarbonate
   - Stay in bath for 15 to 20 minutes.
   - After the bath, remove the residue. Scrub with a loofah sponge or washcloth and rinse the body well.
   - If skin irritation occurs, baths may need to be limited or avoided.
3. Taurine supplements
   - Taurine is a sulfur-bearing amino acid that is also calming and may help lessen unexplained giggling.
   - If your child has an autism disorder, only use taurine under the guidance of a health care practitioner. A subset of children with autism have metabolic disorders and some may be intolerant to taurine.
   - Starting with low doses will reveal any negative responses that should resolve upon cessation.
   - Blood and urine amino acid testing and a metabolic workup (to the degree determined necessary by a health care practitioner) will be helpful in guiding safe use of taurine.

TAURINE TOTAL DAILY GOAL DOSING

AGE	DOSE	FREQUENCY	TOTAL DAILY DOSE FROM ALL SOURCES
2 to 5	150 mg	1 or 2 times per day	300 mg
6 to 10	150 mg	2 times per day	300 mg
11 +	250 mg	2 times per day	500 mg

- Start at half of the lowest recommended dose and increase as tolerated.
- Watch for possible side effects and decrease the dose accordingly.
- If symptoms improve at lower than the goal dose, you may not need to continue to increase the dose.

Low Phenol Diet

If you have eliminated the artificial phenol and salicylate sources and the above measures are not sufficient, you may need to consider a trial elimination of all high-phenol foods. The most common offending foods are apples, grapes (especially red grapes), tomatoes, and cow's milk products. See section 6.2 Low Phenol/Salicylate (Feingold) Diet for additional information and resources.

Section B: Food Intolerances and Elimination of Opioid Food Culprits

Many who have food intolerances exhibit silly behavior and inappropriate laughing and giggling. A full discussion of food intolerances is beyond the scope of this book. More information and resources are available in section 4.17 Digestive Enzymes and section 6.1 Gluten-Free Casein-Free Soy-Free (GFCFSF) Diet.

In short, food proteins, particularly those from milk (casein) and wheat (gluten), may be incompletely digested to peptides and may enter the bloodstream from the intestine via an abnormally permeable intestinal lining (referred to as "leaky gut"). These partially digested protein peptides can potentially cross the blood–brain barrier, negatively affecting brain function, including contributing to mood, attention, and behavior by several mechanisms:

- Blocking neurotransmitter messages
- Creating opiate-like doping effects from gluten (gliadorphin), milk casein (casomorphin), and soy
- Triggering brain inflammation

The most obvious symptom is craving for the food opiate sources (gluten, milk products, and soy). The opiate-like effect is the most common reason for unexplained laughing. The opioid effect can also contribute to language and communication delays, inattention, poor eye contact, irritability, and increased self-stimulating behavior. Effects may occur within an hour of consumption or be delayed up to seventy-two hours.

What to Do and How to Do It

Provided here is a brief summary of two main treatment strategies for food intolerances and the opioid effect.

1. GFCFSF Diet—Elimination Trial: the "gold standard" for treatment
   - The most common problem food proteins are gluten, milk casein, and soy.
   - Your child's body is the best test. Eliminate the food(s) to see whether behavior improves and reintroduce or challenge the body to see whether behavior worsens.
2. Digestive enzymes, including dipeptidyl peptidase-IV (DPP-IV)
   - More efficiently digest gluten, casein, soy and other food proteins, carbohydrates, and fats.
   - Reduce the opioid load due to insufficient DPP-IV enzyme function; this can also "mimic" the diet.

Digestive Enzyme Supplements
See section 4.17 Digestive Enzymes for detailed information on specific enzyme products and dosing.

Section C: Treatment of Intestinal Yeast Overgrowth

Yeast organisms are normal residents of the intestinal tract. Contrary to popular understanding, problematic yeast overgrowth is common in children with a variety of digestive, behavioral, and developmental issues. Treatment may result in notable improvement in a subset of children.

Yeast overgrowth in the intestinal tract can result from inadequate beneficial bacteria that results from antibiotic or steroid use, high sugar intake, and/or poor diet, including inadequate fiber. This can result in physical symptoms such as diaper rashes, oral thrush, skin conditions, intestinal inflammation, and abnormal stools. If yeast toxins are absorbed into the bloodstream through an abnormally permeable intestinal lining, behavioral symptoms can also result. These symptoms can include inattention, anxiety, irritability, silliness, or unexplained laughing.

What to Do and How to Do It
Provided here is a brief summary on treatments for yeast overgrowth. For thorough information and specific guidelines on dosing and side effects, see section 2.18 Yeast Overgrowth, section 4.16 Probiotics, and section 4.6 Biotin.

Main beneficial treatments
- Probiotics (beneficial bacteria)
- Biotin
- Antifungal (anti-yeast) medications or herbs
- Anti-yeast diet

Probiotics
Probiotics are beneficial live microorganisms called the microbiome, found throughout the body, including in the intestinal tract. There are more than 100 trillion good bacteria in the body with 500 to 1,000 different species (forty to fifty of which are main species) in the human gut. They maintain healthy flora, prevent

overgrowth of harmful pathogens and yeast, and also produce healthy nutrients. For a complete listing of probiotic benefits, specific products, and dosing guidelines, see section 4.16 Probiotics and section 2.18 Yeast Overgrowth.

Biotin
Biotin is a water-soluble B vitamin, manufactured in the human digestive tract by healthy flora. Antibiotics depress biotin production, which leads to yeast/fungal overgrowth. Biotin helps keep yeast in a less invasive form, which makes it easier to eradicate. Biotin is one of the safest supplements. It has no toxicity at any level. See section 4.6 The Helper B: Biotin for more information and dosing guidelines.

Antifungal Medications or Herbs
Probiotics help provide beneficial bacteria to the intestinal tract but do not directly kill yeast. To bring yeast levels back down to normal levels, antifungal medications or herbs are used. Probiotics then help maintain good bacterial balance to help prevent yeast overgrowth from recurring.

Antifungal treatments may include herbs or prescription medications. Depending on the amount of yeast present, intestinal symptoms and behavioral side effects from treatment may be significant. Known as "yeast die-off" symptoms, these may include irritability, behavioral regression, and flu-like symptoms. Because of the potential for significant side effects, antifungal treatment should be guided by a health care practitioner based on your child's history and, where possible, specific testing for yeast. See section 2.18 Yeast Overgrowth for additional treatment information.

Anti-Yeast Diet
The anti-yeast diet avoids foods that "feed" yeast: sugars, yeast, starches, fruit juices, refined grains, and processed meats. Sugar is the primary culprit and should be limited or avoided. See section 6.4 Anti-Yeast Diet for detailed references.

▪ *2.16 Skin Problems: Eczema, Dry Skin, and Rashes*
Eczema can be seen alone or in combination with other allergy-related symptoms. Eczema can cause physical symptoms such as itching. Various nutritional deficiencies can contribute to eczema.

Symptoms/signs your child may exhibit
- Eczema, particularly in elbow creases and behind knees
- Generally dry skin
- Keratosis pilaris ("chicken skin" bumps), often on upper arms

Main possible nutritional contributing factors
- Essential fatty acid deficiency
- Zinc deficiency
- Vitamin A deficiency

Skin Problems

- Vitamin D deficiency
- Biotin deficiency
- Inadequate gut flora

DETERMINING WHICH SUPPLEMENTS AND DIET CHANGES MAY BE HELPFUL

IF YOUR CHILD HAS ECZEMA, DRY SKIN, RASHES, AND SOME OF THE FOLLOWING SYMPTOMS	SEE THE APPLICABLE SECTION BELOW	DIETARY AND OTHER RECOMMENDATIONS	OTHER SOURCES OF INFORMATION
Cracking, peeling, and chipping nails Attention problems Cognitive dysfunction Language delays Vision dysfunction Excessive thirst Hard earwax	Section A: Essential Omega-3 Fatty Acids		Chapter 4: section 4.15 Essential Omega-3 Fatty Acids
Picky appetite White lines on nails Frequent illness Language delays Sensory sensitivities Growth delays	Section B: Zinc		Chapter 4: section 4.9 Zinc
Poor eye contact Night blindness Sideways glancing Frequent illness	Section C: Vitamin A		Chapter 4: section 4.1 Vitamin A
Red, scaly cracked "ring around the mouth" Profuse sweating Delayed tooth eruption Bowing legs Bulging forehead "Knobby" knees or ankles Developmental delays	Section D: Vitamin D	Sun exposure, if tolerated	Chapter 4: section 4.2 Vitamin D
Yeast overgrowth Hair loss "Cradle cap" Antibiotic use Coated tongue Diarrhea, gas, bloating	Section E: Biotin and Probiotics		Chapter 2: section 2.18 Yeast Overgrowth Chapter 4: section 4.6 Biotin and section 4.16 Probiotics

Section A: Essential Omega-3 Fatty Acids

Omega-3 fatty acids are critical to immunity, brain, vision, and epithelial health. The skin symptoms are more apparent physically. A lack of sufficient omega-3 fatty acids, especially EPA, can result in eczema, dry skin, and "chicken skin" bumps (keratosis pilaris), which are usually on the upper arms or thighs. Other symptoms include nail cracking, splitting, or peeling, poor hair quality, ADHD, inattention, and poor motor development. Omega-3 fatty acids can help heal skin "from the inside out."

What to Do and How to Do It

Provided here is a brief summary on omega-3 fatty acids. For thorough information and specific guidelines on supplement brands, dosing and side effects, see section 4.15 Essential Omega-3 Fatty Acids.

The best food sources of omega-3 fatty acids are seafood. Those highest in mercury, PCBs, and other toxins include tomalley (crab mustard), farmed fish trout, imported shrimp, and the large "steak" fish such as tuna, bluefish, swordfish, and shark. The safest choices include anchovies, sardines, domestic shrimp, rockfish, and tilapia. For details, see the Environmental Working Group website, www.ewg.org, and the Environmental Defense Fund website, www.edf.org.

Omega-3 supplements for skin conditions
- For skin conditions, we recommend that the EPA amount be equal to or greater than DHA.
- Use only direct fish-source EPA and DHA, which is more efficient than the flaxseed source of ALA.
- Use toxin-free supplements, such as pharmaceutical grade or molecular distillation to remove toxins.
- Vitamins A and D are also helpful to skin. These may be taken separately or together with the omega-3s as cod liver oil.

Types of omega-3 supplements available in capsules, liquids, and chewables
- Cod liver oil (contain varying amounts of vitamins A and D)
- Fish oils with EPA, DHA (most have more EPA than DHA)
- Fish oils higher in DHA (not as helpful for skin issues)
- Vegetarian ALA flaxseed oil (not efficiently converted to EPA, DHA)
- Vegetarian algae-source DHA

The following supplements have higher levels of EPA than DHA
- Nordic Naturals ProOmega or Ultimate Omega with or without D_3
- Carlson Labs Very Finest Fish Oil
- Coromega Squeeze with or without D_3

OMEGA-3 EPA AND DHA TOTAL DAILY GOAL DOSING

AGE	EPA	DHA	FREQUENCY
2 to 5	200 to 400 mg	200 to 400 mg	Daily with food
6 to 10	500 to 650 mg	400 to 500 mg	Daily with food
11 +	500 to 800 mg	500 to 650 mg	Daily with food

If including sources of omega-3 that contain vitamin A, follow the guidelines in section C on vitamin A dosing. Higher doses of the omega-3 fatty acids may be indicated for your child; however, dosing should be determined by a health care practitioner.

Section B: Zinc

Zinc is critical to vitamin A, which is carried in the body by zinc-dependent retinol-binding protein. When zinc is deficient (and therefore vitamin A as well), the skin is vulnerable to a wide range of conditions including eczema, acne, dermatitis, keratosis pilaris (chicken skin), rashes, and hives. Also affected are the epithelial tissues inside the body including the mucosal tissues of the mouth, nasal cavities, sinuses, digestive tract, and more. Zinc deficiency is extremely common in children with autism and is not unusual in children with ADHD.

What to Do and How to Do It

Provided here is a brief summary on zinc. For thorough information and specific guidelines on dosing and side effects, see section 4.9 Zinc.

Zinc supplements
- Well tolerated: gluconates, chelates, citrates, acetates, picolinates, chlorides, and bisglycinates
- Strong taste, needs disguising: sulfates

ZINC TOTAL DAILY GOAL DOSING

AGE	DOSE	FREQUENCY	TOTAL DAILY DOSE FROM ALL SOURCES
2 to 5	5 to 10 mg	1 to 2 times per day	10 to 20 mg
6 to 10	10 mg	2 times per day	20 mg
11 +	10 to 15 mg	2 times per day	20 to 30 mg

For optimal oral absorption, an empty stomach is best, but it may not be feasible if nausea occurs. Large doses can cause gastric discomfort, nausea, and inhibit the digestive enzyme DPP-IV (digests opioids from gluten, casein). In addition:
- Avoid or limit giving zinc at the same time as interfering nutrients: calcium, iron, folate, and phosphorylated nutrients (R5P, P5P, phosphatidyl-choline), although this may not always be feasible.
- Zinc excess can lower copper levels. Copper levels need to be maintained.
- Use the Zinc Tally Taste Test on page 213 for evaluating progress with zinc supplementation.
- Higher doses may be required because of malabsorption, antacid use, the presence of toxic metals, or lab findings. This should be accomplished with a skilled health care practitioner.

Section C: Vitamin A

The most common cause of vitamin A deficiency is zinc deficiency, which is why they share some of the same symptoms. Vitamin A is necessary for the maintenance and repair of epithelial tissue. Deficiency can result in epithelial inflammation, eczema, dermatitis, acne, and the classical vitamin A deficiency symptom—keratosis pilaris. Vitamin A deficiency has been noted in a subset of children with autism.

What to Do and How to Do It

There are differences in the forms and versions of vitamin A with regard to effectiveness on skin conditions.

- Beta-carotene is not the most efficient source of vitamin A for skin conditions.
- Preformed vitamin A is more effective and is found in the following types:
  — Retinoids
  — Micellized vitamin A (water soluble, well-absorbed form)
- Synthetic vitamin A palmitate

VITAMIN A TOTAL DAILY GOAL DOSING

AGE	TOTAL DAILY DOSE FROM ALL SOURCES
2 to 3	1,250 IU
4 to 5	1,250 to 2,500 IU
6 to 10	2,500 to 3,500 IU
11 +	3,500 to 5,000 IU

- Micellized vitamin products absorb more efficiently and are useful in malabsorption.
- Commercially available micellized vitamin A products are usually high dose (5,000 IU). More appropriate strength drops can be made by a compounding pharmacy.
- Zinc is critical for vitamin A transport and utilization. See section B.
- Adequate vitamin D is required when taking vitamin A. See section D.
- Excess vitamin A can result in headaches.
- Higher doses may be required because of malabsorption or lab findings. This should be accomplished with a health care practitioner.

Section D: Vitamin D

Vitamin D deficiency is very common. Vitamin D is important for skin health and immunity. Deficiencies result in poor skin health and dry, scaly cracked lips. Risk factors for the development of vitamin D deficiency include inadequate sun exposure (or use of sunblock), darker skin pigmentation, obesity, breast feeding, low dietary intake, and fat malabsorption.

Provided here is a brief summary on vitamin D. For thorough information and specific guidelines on dosing and side effects, see section 4.2 Vitamin D.

What to Do and How to Do It

The forms and versions of vitamin D supplements are varied. It is important to understand the differences.

- Vitamin D_3 (cholecalciferol) is available in capsules, tablets, and liquids.
- The micellized version of vitamin D_3 is a water-soluble form that is well absorbed and especially useful in malabsorption conditions.
- Vitamin D_3 is the best form to use for supplementation.

Skin Problems

- Vitamin D_2 (ergocalciferol) converts to vitamin D_3 and is less effective.
- The oil and micellized forms are preferred over the dry forms.

VITAMIN D TOTAL DAILY GOAL DOSING

AGE	TOTAL DAILY DOSE FROM ALL SOURCES	FREQUENCY
2 to 5	400 to 600 IU	Daily
6 to 10	600 to 800 IU	Daily
11 +	800 to 2,000 IU	Daily

- The total daily dose includes all sources such as vitamin D from cod liver oil and multiple vitamins.
- Do blood testing (25-hydroxy vitamin D) to guide dosing. The optimal goal level is 60 to 80 ng/mL.
- Adequate vitamin A intake must be maintained. See the vitamin A recommendations in section C.
- Higher doses may be required because of malabsorption or lab findings. This should be accomplished with a health care practitioner.

Section E: Biotin and Probiotics

Biotin is a water-soluble B vitamin, manufactured in the human digestive tract by healthy flora. Antibiotics depress biotin production, which leads to yeast and fungal overgrowth and skin conditions, especially eczema, rashes, seborrheic dermatitis, and "cradle cap." Biotin is one of the safest supplements. It has no toxicity at any level.

Provided here is a brief summary on biotin. For thorough information and specific guidelines on dosing and side effects, see section 4.6 Biotin.

BIOTIN TOTAL DAILY GOAL DOSING

AGE	DOSE	FREQUENCY
2 to 5	500 mcg to 5 mg	Daily
6 to 10	5 mg	Daily
11 +	5 to 10 mg	Daily

- Supplementation can range from 100 mcg to 50 mg depending upon the extent of enzyme defects in biotin metabolism.
- For doses beyond 10 mg, include magnesium supplementation.
- Higher doses should be accomplished only under the guidance of a health care practitioner.

Probiotics

Probiotics are beneficial live microorganisms called the microbiome, found throughout the body including in the intestinal tract. There are more than 100 trillion good bacteria in the body with 500 to 1,000 different species (forty to fifty of which are main species) in the human gut. In addition to maintaining healthy digestion, gut milieu, stools, and immunity, they are important in skin health.

What to Do and How to Do It

Provided here is a summary on probiotics. For more thorough information, see section 4.16 Probiotics.

Probiotic supplements
- May be in single strain to multistrain cultures (*Lactobacillus, Bifidobacteria, Streptococcus, Saccharomyces*)
- Should contain live strains, be stored in freezers prior to use, be shipped on ice, and be stored in refrigerator once opened
- Should be hypoallergenic (no milk, casein, gluten, soy, corn, or artificial additives)

Types of supplements
- *Bifidus infantis* or bifido complexes (for infants)
- *Lactobacillus acidophilus*
- *Lactobacillus/Bifidus* combinations
- Expanded combinations with multiple strains
- *Saccharomyces boulardii* (a beneficial yeast)

PROBIOTIC TOTAL DAILY GOAL DOSING

AGE	DOSE IN CFUS	FREQUENCY *TAKE WITH FOOD*
1 to 2	1 to 5 billion	Begin with single *Bifidobacteria* product. Expand to mixed cultures for infants, especially if formula fed.
3 to 5	5 to 10 billion	In 2 divided doses
6 to 10	10 to 20 billion	In 2 divided doses
11 +	10 to 50 billion	In 2 divided doses

- Start low and increase slowly to try to avoid die-off side effects.
  - For products with 5 to 10 billion bacteria, start with one-quarter to one-half capsule once daily and increase by one-quarter to one-half capsule every two to three days until on goal dose or die-off symptoms begin to develop.
  - For higher dose probiotics, start with one-quarter capsule and increase by one-quarter capsule every two to three days.
- Probiotics are best taken with mild-temperature food and can also be taken on an empty stomach.
- If taking antibiotics, wait at least one hour to give probiotics.
- Consult with a health care practitioner for guidance in using higher doses of probiotics.

If problems persist and symptoms suggest yeast overgrowth, the anti-yeast diet should be considered. See section 6.4 Anti-Yeast Diet.

Skin Problems

◼ 2.17 *Sleep Difficulties*

As parents well know, sleep problems are extremely common in children with autism. Sleep can also be a challenge at times for children with ADHD, anxiety, or other behavioral or developmental issues. Improving sleep improves not only the health and functioning of the child, but of the entire family. If a child is not sleeping, no one is sleeping.

Symptoms/signs your child may exhibit
- Difficulty falling asleep
- Restless sleep
- Night waking

Main possible contributing nutritional factors
- Magnesium deficiency
- Need for melatonin
- Need for GABA
- Low serotonin
- Elevated mid-sleep cortisol
- Histamine from allergies

DETERMINING WHICH SUPPLEMENTS AND DIET CHANGES MAY BE HELPFUL

IF YOUR CHILD HAS SLEEP DIFFICULTIES AND SOME OF THE FOLLOWING SYMPTOMS	SEE THE APPLICABLE SECTION BELOW	DIETARY AND OTHER RECOMMENDATIONS	OTHER SOURCES OF INFORMATION
Restless sleep Nightmares Night terrors Sound sensitivity Moodiness Anxiety Excessive sighing Easy startle	Section A: Magnesium		Chapter 4: section 4.8 Magnesium and Calcium
Trouble falling asleep	Section B: Melatonin	Dark room for sleep	
Anxiety: • Interfering with falling asleep • Causing mid-sleep awakening	Section C: GABA		Chapter 4: section 4.11 GABA and Theanine
Night waking	Section D: Ashwagandha		
Allergy symptoms: • Runny nose • Sneezing • Itchy eyes or nose • Dark circles under eyes ("allergic shiners") • Eczema/atopic dermatitis, hives • Food-induced rash around the mouth • Food-induced redness around the anus	Section E: Histamine Reduction	Elimination of allergy sources	Chapter 2: section 2.1 Allergies

Section A: Magnesium

Magnesium deficiency can lead to neuromuscular excitability, which results in poor sleep and/or restless sleep. Magnesium has calming effects on the nervous system and can improve both the duration and quality of sleep. Magnesium is a common nutritional deficiency in children with ADHD or autism. It is also a common deficiency in the general population.

What to Do and How to Do It
Provided here is a brief summary on magnesium. For thorough information and specific guidelines on dosing, see section 4.8 Magnesium and Calcium.

Magnesium supplements
- Gentle (less laxative) stool effect: chelates, aspartates, glycinates, gluconates, and bisglycinates
- Laxative stool effect: citrates, chlorides, and sulfates

MAGNESIUM TOTAL DAILY GOAL DOSING

AGE	DOSE	FREQUENCY	TOTAL DAILY DOSE FROM ALL SOURCES
2 to 5	100 mg	1 or 2 times per day	200 mg
6 to 10	100 mg	2 or 3 times per day	300 mg
11 +	100 to 150 mg	2 or 3 times per day	450 mg

- Start at one-quarter to one-half of the recommended dose and increase the dose gradually every one to two days.
- Magnesium can cause loose stools or diarrhea, which then can deplete magnesium.
- Watch for possible side effects and decrease the dose accordingly.
- If symptoms improve at lower than the goal dose, you may not need to continue to increase the dose.
- For higher-than-recommended doses, consult with a health care practitioner.

Calcium
Make sure calcium intake, either through diet or supplement, is adequate. Magnesium intake can lower calcium, and calcium intake can lower magnesium. It is important to have balance. If your child is not getting sufficient calcium from diet, a calcium supplement is indicated.

CALCIUM TOTAL DAILY GOAL DOSING

AGE	DOSE	FREQUENCY	TOTAL DAILY DOSE FROM ALL SOURCES
2 to 5	250 mg	2 times per day	500 mg
6 to 10	250 mg	3 times per day	750 mg
11 +	500 to 600 mg	2 times per day	1,000 to 1,200 mg

Sleep Difficulties

Section B: Melatonin

Melatonin is a hormone produced by the pineal gland located in the brain. It is manufactured from tryptophan, which converts to serotonin and on to melatonin. Melatonin is stored during the day and released at night when there is a lack of light exposure for a length of time. It tells the body it is time to go to sleep. If your child is exposed to light during the night, either through night waking or not sleeping in a dark enough room, the normal melatonin cycle may be disrupted. Melatonin helps maintain a healthy sleep cycle. Time-release forms may help with staying asleep. However, night waking is not usually due to low melatonin, and other factors may need to be considered (see section D, Ashwagandha, and section E, Histamine Reduction, for additional information).

What to Do and How to Do It

Melatonin is commercially available as liquid, chewable tablets, or capsules. It can also be compounded into a transdermal lotion. Melatonin takes thirty to sixty minutes to have an effect. Therefore, the dose should be given thirty to sixty minutes before you would like your child to be asleep.

The time of sleep onset can vary from person to person, and you will learn how quickly melatonin works for your child. If your child wakes, you can give one additional dose of melatonin. We recommend not giving this dose after 4 a.m., as there is then a chance of morning sluggishness or sleepiness.

MELATONIN TOTAL DAILY GOAL DOSING

AGE	DOSE	FREQUENCY
2 to 5	0.5 to 1 mg	30 to 60 minutes before bedtime
6 to 10	1 to 3 mg	30 to 60 minutes before bedtime
11 +	1 to 4 mg	30 to 60 minutes before bedtime

We recommend starting with 1 mg and increasing by 1 mg every two nights until restful sleep is achieved or until the maximum recommended dose is achieved. For two- to three-year-old children, start with 0.5 mg and increase by 0.5 mg every two nights. Doses higher than those listed above may be needed in some cases; however, we recommend guidance by a health care practitioner.

If your child wakes at night, you can give an additional dose of melatonin. You may need to use the same dose you gave at bedtime. However, sometimes a lower dose is sufficient to get a child to return to sleep. We would therefore recommend starting with the lower end of the recommended dosing range for your child's age and increasing the dose gradually until you find the dose necessary to help your child return to sleep.

It is obviously not ideal for your child (or for you) to be waking nightly to get a second dose of melatonin. Night waking may indicate a different issue, such as an early cortisol peak, and may require an additional or different treatment. See section D on ashwagandha for more details.

What Side Effects Should I Watch for?
Side effects from melatonin are rare. The main side effect of melatonin is daytime sleepiness if a dose is given after 4 a.m. There are some individuals who have an opposite reaction and are more alert. This is not common.

What Else Should I Know?
Melatonin may be safely taken for extended periods of time. For children with chronic sleep difficulties, nightly use is recommended initially to help reestablish consistent sleep. This may help reestablish a child's own normal melatonin cycle. For less chronic conditions, melatonin may only need to be used for shorter periods or on an as-needed basis. After a period of extended use, it is worth stopping melatonin for a night or two to see whether it is still needed. We would recommend doing this trial on a weekend when you and your child can catch up on sleep during the day if needed.

Darkness is key to melatonin release. If you can't keep the bedroom dark enough that you can't see your hand in front of your face, consider getting blackout shades.

Section C: GABA

GABA is a calming amino acid and inhibitory neurotransmitter. It is helpful in treating anxiety and may help with sleep problems when anxiety prevents going to sleep and/or there is mid-sleep anxiety-induced awakening.

What to Do and How to Do It
Provided here is a brief summary on GABA. For thorough information and specific guidelines on dosing, see section 4.11 GABA and Theanine.

- GABA is best absorbed on an empty stomach, which may not be feasible. It may be taken with food.
- GABA's beneficial effects may affect dosing of medications used for ADHD, anxiety, and seizures. Do not add GABA without discussing with your child's prescribing physician.
- GABA should not be used if the child is already taking a medication that increases or potentially affects GABA, such as benzodiazepines, barbiturates, narcotics, and gabapentin.
- GABA, especially at higher doses, should only be used under the guidance of a health care health care practitioner.
- Side effects can include lethargy, excitability, and irritability.

GABA TOTAL DAILY GOAL DOSING

AGE	DOSE	FREQUENCY	TOTAL DAILY DOSE FROM ALL SOURCES
2 to 5	25 to 50 mg	2 times per day (breakfast and dinner)	50 to 100 mg
6 to 10	50 to 100 mg	2 times per day (breakfast and dinner)	100 to 200 mg
11 +	250 mg	1 or 2 times per day (breakfast and dinner)	250 to 500 mg

Sleep Difficulties

Section D: Ashwagandha

Night waking is often due to an early peak of a hormone known as cortisol. Cortisol is a hormone produced by the adrenal gland. The circadian rhythm of cortisol is regulated by the sleep–wake cycle. Cortisol secretion normally has a steep increase in the morning, peaking at approximately 8 a.m., followed by a gradual tapering off until midnight. Cortisol is an alerting hormone. When an individual experiences chronic stress, the adrenal glands can become fatigued and dysregulated. This results in the cortisol peak occurring earlier and earlier during the night, resulting in night waking. When night waking is due to cortisol, children are often very alert and ready to start their day.

Ashwagandha is an herb that helps nourish and re-regulate the adrenal glands. In so doing, it helps move the cortisol peak back to its normal time. Ashwagandha also has anti-anxiety benefits.

What to Do and How to Do It

Ashwagandha can have a very wide dosing range. We recommend that you start at a low dose and increase the dose gradually. It may take a couple of weeks at a stable dose to see the full benefit. For young children who cannot swallow pills, you may need to have ashwagandha compounded into a liquid to allow for appropriate dosing. Older children and adolescents may be able to use commercially available tablets or capsules.

Dosing guidelines are difficult to give for the tincture forms of ashwagandha. Herbal tinctures often do not provide milligram amounts. For children who cannot swallow tablets or capsules, get ashwagandha dosing guidelines from your child's health care practitioner who may be familiar with specific ashwagandha products. Compounding pharmacists may also be able to provide guidance.

For children who can swallow pills, general guidelines are offered below.

ASHWAGANDHA TOTAL DAILY GOAL DOSING

AGE	DOSE	FREQUENCY
2 to 5	100 mg	At bedtime
6 to 10	200 mg	At bedtime
11 +	200 to 400 mg	At bedtime

What Side Effects Should I Watch for?

Side effects from ashwagandha are uncommon. Daytime sedation is very rare. Side *benefits* of ashwagandha can be a decrease in anxiety and an improvement in energy levels.

What Else Should I Know?

It is okay to take both melatonin and ashwagandha together. Many children need both because the two supplements address different issues. If your child wakes before 4 a.m., the same dose of ashwagandha can be repeated.

Section E: Histamine Reduction

Histamine is a chemical released in individuals who have allergies and is usually associated with a runny nose, nasal congestion, postnasal drip, itchy eyes or nose, and skin rashes. Some of histamine's negative effects are caused by histamine binding to cells, which then result in these symptoms. Histamine can have an alerting effect in the brain that can disrupt sleep. Suspect histamine as a contributing factor if your child's sleep worsens during allergy season or when he or she has physical symptoms suggestive of allergies.

What to Do and How to Do It
Provided here is a brief summary on histamine. For thorough information and specific guidelines on dosing and side effects, see section 2.1 Allergies.

Basic strategies
1. Removing the triggers for allergies
   • Inhalants (e.g., grass, trees, pollen, mold, animal danders)
   • Food that causes type I IgE histamine-releasing allergies
2. Using antihistamine medications. Antihistamine medications are often recommended for short periods of time to "break the cycle" in the hopes of allowing a regular sleep cycle to return. We would not recommend this approach beyond a couple of nights.
3. Taking supplements that reduce histamine release.

Antihistamines affect REM sleep ("dream sleep"), which is the most restorative part of the sleep cycle, so the sleep your child gets on antihistamines is not good-quality sleep. Quercetin, pantothenic acid, and Vitamin C are natural antihistamines and can result in better-quality sleep.

Recent studies through the NIH are also finding decreased REM sleep in a subset of children with autism.

SUPPLEMENTS THAT REDUCE HISTAMINE RELEASE

SUPPLEMENT	DESCRIPTION	QUALITIES	AGE	DAILY DOSE	TOTAL DAILY DOSE
Quercetin	Plant flavonol Anti-inflammatory	Bright yellow, tasteless. Mix in juice, fruit sauce.	2 to 5 6 to 10 11 +	250 mg 2 times per day 500 mg 2 times per day 500 mg 2 times per day	500 mg 1,000 mg 1,000 mg
Pantothenic acid (vitamin B$_5$)	Water soluble B vitamin Nontoxic	Mix in food, juice, smoothies.	2 to 5 6 to 10 11 +	100 to 250 mg per day 250 mg 2 or 3 times per day 500 mg 2 times per day	250 mg 750 mg 1,000 mg
Vitamin C (ascorbic acid)	Water soluble Nontoxic Excess causes loose stools	Mix in food, juice, smoothies.	2 to 5 6 to 10 11 +	100 to 250 mg per day 250 mg 2 or 3 times per day 500 mg 2 times per day	250 mg 750 mg 1,000 mg

• Lower doses can be used for maintenance and reducing allergy potential.
• All three of the supplements may be taken together

Sleep Difficulties

■ 2.18 *Yeast Overgrowth*

Yeast organisms are normal residents of the intestinal tract. Contrary to popular understanding, problematic yeast overgrowth is common in children with a variety of digestive, behavioral, and developmental issues. Treatment may result in notable improvement in a subset of children.

When present in normal amounts along with adequate numbers of beneficial bacteria, yeast does not cause a problem. When yeast is present in an excessive amount, it can:

1. Cause intestinal inflammation, which may be a trigger for systemic (total body) inflammation, including inflammation of the brain, particularly in children with autism spectrum disorders.
2. Affect intestinal permeability (referred to as "leaky gut"), which allows unwanted molecules (such as partially digested food proteins or opiate-like peptides) to cross from the intestine into the bloodstream.
3. Produce toxic chemicals, which can aggravate the intestinal lining and subsequently enter the bloodstream. If these toxins reach the brain, they can adversely affect brain function.
4. Interfere with the DPP-IV enzyme, which helps digest opiate-like peptides from casein or gluten.

Symptoms/signs your child may exhibit
- Chronic or recurrent diaper rashes
- Oral thrush (white plaques on tongue or inside of cheeks)
- Loose or smelly stools
- Skin rashes, eczema, dermatitis
- Silly behavior or unexplained giggling
- Poor attention

Main possible contributing factors
- Recurrent use of antibiotics and/or steroids
- Poor fiber intake
- High sugar diet

Main beneficial treatments
- Probiotics ("beneficial" bacteria) (See section A)
- Biotin (See section B)
- Antifungal (anti-yeast) medications or herbs (See section C)
- Anti-yeast diet (See section D)

Section A: Probiotics

Probiotics are beneficial live microorganisms called the microbiome, found throughout the body, including the intestinal tract. There are more than 100 trillion good bacteria in the body with 500 to 1,000 different species (forty to fifty of which are main species) in the human gut. These beneficial bacteria serve many important functions including maintaining healthy flora, preventing overgrowth of harmful pathogens and yeast, and producing healthy nutrients. For a complete listing of probiotic benefits, see section 4.16 Probiotics.

What to Do and How to Do It
Provided here is a summary on probiotics. For more thorough information on products and dosing, see section 4.16 Probiotics.

Probiotic supplements
- May be in single strain to multistrain cultures (*Lactobacillus, Bifidobacteria, Streptococcus,* and *Saccharomyces*)
- Should contain live strains, be stored in freezers prior to use, be shipped on ice, and be stored in the refrigerator during use
- Should be hypoallergenic (no milk, casein, gluten, soy, corn, or artificial additives)

Types of supplements
- *Bifidus infantis* or bifido complexes (for infants)
- *Lactobacillus acidophilus*
- *Lactobacillus/Bifidus* combinations
- Expanded combinations with multiple strains
- *Saccharomyces boulardii* (a "beneficial" yeast)

PROBIOTIC TOTAL DAILY GOAL DOSING

AGE	DOSE IN CFUS	FREQUENCY (TAKE WITH FOOD)
1 to 2	1 to 5 billion	Begin with single *Bifidobacteria* product. Expand to mixed cultures for infants, especially if formula fed.
3 to 5	5 to 10 billion	In 2 divided doses
6 to 10	10 to 20 billion	In 2 divided doses
11 +	10 to 50 billion	In 2 divided doses

- Start low and increase slowly to try to avoid die-off side effects.
  - For products with 5 to 10 billion bacteria, start with one-quarter to one-half capsule once daily and increase by one-quarter to one-half capsule every two to three days until on goal dose or die-off symptoms develop.
  - For higher dose probiotics, start with one-quarter capsule and increase by one-quarter capsule every two to three days.
- Probiotics are best taken with mild-temperature food and can also be taken on an empty stomach.
- If taking antibiotics, wait at least one hour to give probiotics.
- Consult with a health care practitioner for guidance in increasing the dose.

Yeast Overgrowth

Section B: Biotin

Biotin is a water-soluble B vitamin, manufactured in the human digestive tract by healthy flora. Antibiotics depress biotin production, which leads to yeast and fungal overgrowth. Biotin helps keep yeast in a less invasive form, which makes it easier to eradicate. Biotin is one of the safest supplements. It has no toxicity at any level.

What to Do and How to Do It
Provided here is a brief summary on biotin. For thorough information, see section 4.6 Biotin.

BIOTIN TOTAL DAILY GOAL DOSING

AGE	DOSE	FREQUENCY
2 to 5	500 mcg to 5 mg	Daily
6 to 10	5 mg	Daily
11 +	5 to 10 mg	Daily

- Supplementation can range from 100 mcg to 50 mg depending upon the extent of enzyme defects in biotin metabolism.
- For doses beyond 10 mg, it is important to include magnesium supplementation.
- Higher doses should be accomplished only under the guidance of a health care practitioner.

Section C: Antifungal Medications or Herbs

Probiotics help provide beneficial bacteria to the intestinal tract but do not directly kill yeast. To bring yeast levels back down to normal levels, antifungal medications or herbs are used. Probiotics then help maintain good bacterial balance to help prevent yeast overgrowth from recurring.

Excessive yeast can cause obvious physical symptoms such as diaper rashes, oral thrush, or abnormal stools. However, yeast toxins, if absorbed into the bloodstream through an abnormally permeable intestinal lining, can also affect behavior. It is not unusual to see silly behavior or unexplained giggling from these yeast-generated toxins. The yeast itself does not enter the bloodstream, just its toxins. It is possible, and not uncommon, to have behavioral issues from yeast overgrowth without any obvious physical symptoms.

What to Do and How to Do It
We would recommend that specific antifungal treatments be guided by a health care practitioner. Urine testing for yeast toxins and/or stool testing for culturing of bacteria and yeast are recommended to determine whether your child has an imbalance, to what degree, and what antifungal treatments are most likely to effective. Depending on the amount of yeast overgrowth present, intestinal symptoms and behavioral side effects to yeast treatment can be signifi-

cant. If a substantial number of yeast are killed, they will release a large amount of toxins. If more toxins are generated than can be adequately excreted through the stool in a timely fashion, the toxins will be absorbed into the bloodstream and behavioral side effects can occur. These are commonly referred to as "yeast die-off" effects. Symptoms can range from mild irritability to major behavioral regression. Knowing your child's degree of yeast burden helps guide the choice, type, and dosing of antifungal medications or herbs.

Yeast treatments include:
- Medications (e.g., Nystatin, Diflucan)
- Herbs (e.g., olive leaf extract, barberry, goldenseal, neem, grapefruit seed extract, pau d'arco, allicin/garlic, oregano oil)

What Else Should I Know?
Yeast treatment usually requires more than one round of treatment. Yeast can mutate and become resistant to medications or herbs. Health care practitioners have different approaches to treating yeast, with various agents and durations of treatment. As a general rule, we prefer to start treating yeast with a gentle antifungal first, then progressing to stronger or more broad-spectrum antifungals later. We have found this allows for better tolerance of treatment.

Some advocate starting with a strong antifungal and trying to tolerate the behavioral side effects, to get rid of the yeast more quickly. We would argue against that approach as it may result in flooding a developing brain with excessive toxins, which we do not feel is healthy, even in the short term. In addition, if your child has significant yeast die-off side effects, he or she will not be available for learning during that time. The goal should be the most aggressive yeast treatment tolerated, one step shy of causing significant side effects. Whatever antifungal is chosen, start with a low dose and increase gradually to lessen the chance of yeast die-off.

It is also important for your child to have daily stools during yeast treatment, to optimize elimination of the generated yeast toxins. If constipation is an issue, consider adding magnesium citrate to achieve daily stools. See section 4.8 Magnesium and Calcium.

Section D: Anti-Yeast Diet
The anti-yeast diet avoids foods that "feed" yeast overgrowth: sugars, yeast, starches, fruit juices, refined grains, and processed meats. Sugar is the primary culprit and should be limited or avoided. In general, we prefer to try the treatments listed above first, and recommend more restrictive diet changes primarily for persistent yeast that is resistant to treatment. See section 6.4 Anti-Yeast/Anti-*Candida* Diet for additional information and resources.

Yeast Overgrowth

CHAPTER 3

Getting to Know the Landscape: The Primary Systems, Mechanisms, and Epigenetics

Every child with ADHD or autism is unique in how the condition each one experiences manifests itself. A cluster of similarities, however, has evolved in the systems affected, the biochemical mechanisms, and the impact of environment on genetics. The symptoms presented in the first half of this book are not the causes of the diagnostic labels, rather they are the outward indicators of one or more underlying disorders, deficiencies, and imbalances.

Understanding the fundamental physiology, biochemistry, and genomics can help both health care providers and families better understand some of the important pieces of the puzzle we label "autism." In ADHD, many of the same systems and metabolic mechanisms are involved, but to a lesser degree.

Admittedly, these concepts can be complex for anyone. We have endeavored to give you an overview that provides some clarity and direction in your journey with your child, in addition to many excellent references to expand your knowledge. The more thoroughly you understand these concepts, the more you can understand your child's condition, and the more effectively you can collaborate with his or her health care practitioners toward improvement.

■ 3.1 Negotiating through the Territory: The Four Primary Systems

▶ A. THE GASTROINTESTINAL (GI) SYSTEM

Although the gastrointestinal system and the brain may be physically distant from each other, they are functionally interconnected, sharing the same neurotransmitters. Problems in the brain affect the bowel and conversely, problems in the bowel affect the brain. Improving intestinal health can therefore potentially improve brain function. Studies suggest that 50 to 70 percent of children with autism have GI issues. Children with ADHD may also have some of these issues, though typically with less frequency and severity.

This section focuses on how digestive system problems can affect the brain. This can potentially occur through many mechanisms, including:

- Altered intestinal permeability ("leaky gut")
- Poor/incomplete digestion of food proteins (especially casein, gluten, and soy)
- Bacterial dysbiosis and intestinal yeast overgrowth
- Intestinal inflammation
- Celiac disease

Altered Intestinal Permeability ("Leaky Gut")

In the small intestine, foods are digested and nutrients absorbed. The lining of the intestine is designed to let small molecules, such as nutrients, cross into the bloodstream and prevent larger molecules, such as partially digested food proteins and toxins from entering. Many conditions can alter this permeability by loosening the junctions between the intestinal cells such as nutrient deficiencies, immune deficiency, inflammation, celiac disease, dysbiosis, toxins, specific medications, and chronic stress. This "leakiness" allows molecules to enter the bloodstream, with adverse consequences such as systemic inflammation, immune reactions, and/or negative effects on brain function.

Treatment of "leaky gut" includes eliminating the causes and providing supportive treatments such as: digestive enzymes, omega-3 fatty acids, vitamin A, zinc, probiotics, glutamine, anti-inflammatory nutrients, and aloe vera.

Poor Food Digestion

Digestion begins in the brain; the thought, sight, or smell of food signals the digestive tract to prepare for food. From the mouth, food moves into the stomach for digestion, and on to the small intestine where more than 90 percent of nutrient absorption occurs. What remains of undigested food passes into the colon for preparation for elimination.

For children with ADHD, autism, and other behavioral and developmental disorders, inadequate digestion of food proteins, particularly casein, gluten, and soy, can contribute to physical and behavioral symptoms. Proteins consist of chains of amino acids. During digestion, these chains are broken down into smaller chains of amino acids called peptides, which are then more fully digested to individual amino acids. These amino acids are then absorbed for use by the body.

If digestion is incomplete and the gut is too permeable, partially digested peptide chains can "leak" into the bloodstream. These peptides can trigger immune reactions and also potentially cross the blood–brain barrier and disrupt optimal brain functioning. In individuals with autism, some of the peptide molecules have an opiate- or morphine-like structure. These opiates can occur with casein, gluten, and probably soy, and have an adverse effect on brain function, resulting in symptoms such as silliness or inappropriate laughing, food cravings, acting as if "in a fog," or inattention. Treatment of poor food digestion can include dietary changes, such as eliminating the opioid sources, and the use of digestive enzymes.

The Gastrointestinal (GI) System

Bacterial Dysbiosis and Intestinal Yeast Overgrowth

The intestine is home to trillions of beneficial bacteria. Yeast organisms, which are normal residents of the digestive tract, can overgrow and become problematic when bacterial balance is disrupted by culprits such as antibiotics. This can result in many problems, such as:

- Loss of the myriad benefits from adequate beneficial bacteria (see section 4.16 Probiotics)
- Excessive toxins from yeast or *Clostridia* overgrowth. In the presence of a "leaky gut," these toxins can enter the bloodstream, potentially interfering with brain function. Yeast toxins also inhibit the functioning of the DPP-IV enzyme, which helps digest opiate-like peptides.
- Inflammation of the gastrointestinal tract

Treatments involve probiotics (beneficial bacteria) and antifungal or antibacterial medications or herbs. Dietary changes may also be beneficial (see section 2.18 Yeast Overgrowth).

Intestinal Inflammation

Intestinal inflammation can result from insufficient beneficial bacteria, intestinal pathogens, toxins, food reactions, specific medications, and autoimmunity. Inflammatory bowel disease has been found in a subset of children with autism. This can then trigger more systemic (total body) inflammation, including the brain. Autopsy studies have shown chronic brain inflammation in individuals with autism. Treatment includes identification and correction of the factors triggering inflammation. Use of supplements with anti-inflammatory effects (e.g., quercetin, curcumin) can be helpful.

Celiac Disease

Celiac disease is an autoimmune reaction to gluten. The body inappropriately reacts to gluten, causing an immune attack that damages the small intestinal lining. Intestinal permeability increases and the finger-like projections (villi) of this lining become flattened, resulting in poor nutrient absorption. Celiac disease can result in intestinal, behavioral, skin, and/or neurological symptoms. We recommend that celiac testing be done prior to embarking on a gluten-free diet, because gluten exposure is needed for the blood test to be accurate. The current treatment for celiac disease is a lifelong, strict elimination of gluten.

Clinical Gastrointestinal (GI) Conditions

Digestive conditions can cause physical discomfort. Less recognized is that they can also trigger behavioral problems. Digestive problems in children with ADHD or autism should be taken seriously and not dismissed as simply part of their behavioral diagnosis. They should be evaluated and treated with the same thoroughness as they would in children without these behavioral and developmental disorders.

If any of the following conditions persist, consult your child's physician:

Gastroesophageal reflux disease (GERD). Gastroesophageal reflux is not uncommon in children with autism. In reflux, food comes back up from the stomach into the esophagus or mouth. Symptoms can include burping, coughing, effortless vomiting/regurgitation, and/or heartburn. Although verbal children may be able to describe what is happening, nonverbal children may only show behavioral symptoms. Because reflux symptoms are worse when lying down, the condition should be suspected if there is severe resistance to going to sleep or frequent night waking with or without apparent discomfort. Pain from reflux symptoms may also lead to decreased appetites and self-injurious behaviors. Treatment of reflux can include positioning (e.g., staying upright for an hour after eating), supplements (e.g., calcium given after meals), or acid-suppressing medications. Additional interventions include treating other factors that can aggravate reflux such as constipation and food reactions, especially to cow's milk products.

Constipation. Constipation, a common problem in children, refers to either infrequent stools or hard, difficult-to-pass stools. Stools should be formed but soft and easy to pass and occur on a daily basis. When this does not occur, there can be many adverse consequences including:
- Physical discomfort, from retained stool, gas, or bloating
- Urinary frequency, incontinence, or bedwetting, from stool pressing on the bladder
- Behavioral worsening, from inadequate excretion of toxins. Children's behavior often worsens when they are constipated and improves after bowel movements.
- Worsened reflux symptoms

Constipation may be treated with nutritional supplements and/or medications. (See section 2.6 Constipation for detailed nutritional approaches.) Depending on the degree of constipation, more aggressive measures (e.g., abdominal X-rays to look for impaction, use of enemas, or high-dose laxatives) may be needed initially before maintenance with nutritional supplements can be effective.

Diarrhea. Children can develop diarrhea for reasons ranging from temporary responses to illness, infections, and food reactions, to inflammatory bowel conditions. See section 2.7 Diarrhea for more details.

Abdominal pain, distention, or bloating. These symptoms can be signs of benign, temporary processes (such as transient constipation) or more significant disorders (such as inflammatory bowel disease or a blockage).

Food allergies. A subset of children have true food allergies. Often this is obvious, with clear reactions to specific foods (e.g., hives, respiratory distress). However, sometimes food allergies are more subtle and may manifest as poor eating or nonspecific discomfort. Depending on the severity of symptoms, an evaluation by an allergist or gastroenterologist may be indicated.

Food sensitivities and intolerances. Food sensitivities can include reactions to components in foods (e.g., phenols, salicylates, phenylalanine, gluten, casein, disaccharides, oxalates) and also when incompletely digested food proteins (peptides) enter the bloodstream via a "leaky gut." Peptides from gluten (glia-

The Gastrointestinal (GI) System

dorphin) and casein (casomorphin) can have opiate-like reactions. Other food reactions can trigger immunoglobulin G (IgG) antibodies, which are different from IgE antibodies seen in traditional allergies. IgG reactions can occur immediately or up to seventy-two hours after ingestion of the food culprit causing physical and/or behavioral reactions. A detailed discussion is beyond the scope of this book. Refer to our first book, *The Kid-Friendly ADHD & Autism Cookbook*, for more information.

▶ B. ENERGY METABOLISM AND MITOCHONDRIA

From food breakdown products (e.g., amino acids, glucose, fatty acids), cells generate their own energy molecules for all of their reactions and functions. This process occurs in every cell within mitochondria, the energy-generating machinery necessary for life. A subset of children with autism have problems with mitochondrial function resulting in physical and behavioral symptoms due to insufficient energy availability.

Energy Metabolism Problems
Many metabolic processes require enzymes to process molecules so that they can be further used or eliminated. If these enzymes are absent or not functioning optimally, toxic substances can accumulate and the manufacturing of needed compounds can be impaired.

Complete absence of enzymes is rare. However, it is possible to have less than optimal function of enzymes, either because of inefficiencies or lack of necessary nutritional cofactors. Enzymes require certain nutrients for optimal function. Many require zinc, magnesium, and B vitamins. More than 300 reactions require magnesium, and more than 200 reactions require zinc. Poor dietary intake or poor absorption of nutrients can result in deficiencies of important cofactors. Toxic insults may also damage important enzymes. Children with autism often have weaknesses in their detoxification systems allowing toxins to accumulate, resulting in damage. Medications, such as seizure medications, may deplete needed nutrients (e.g., carnitine). Resulting symptoms may include poor endurance; low muscle tone; and cognitive, focus, and learning issues.

Consider a traffic jam analogy: When an enzyme is completely absent, it is as if a portion of the road was completely destroyed. The resulting traffic jam is severe and you can't get where you need to go. When an enzyme is partially deficient or lacking necessary nutrients, it is like driving on a road that has some of the lanes blocked. The resulting traffic jam is less severe and you can still eventually reach your destination. When molecules "back up," they can interfere with chemical processes. This can result in a variety of clinical symptoms (see the symptom list below). Interventions include providing needed nutrients or, in more severe cases, completely avoiding the food or substance that can't be metabolized. Both approaches relieve the traffic jams.

Symptoms and Strategies

Clinical symptoms suggestive of metabolic or mitochondrial disorders can include:

- Unusual lethargy, vomiting, or limpness in response to illness or fasting
- Unusual odors in urine or sweat
- Poor endurance or easy fatigue
- Hypotonia (low muscle tone)
- Developmental or neurological regression with illness
- Repeated developmental regressions
- Uncontrolled seizures
- Failure to thrive

If your child has any of these symptoms, please discuss them with his or her doctor. Nutrients potentially helpful in metabolic or mitochondrial disorders or dysfunctions include B vitamins, particularly folinic acid and B_{12}, zinc, magnesium, biotin, carnitine, and coenzyme Q_{10}. A thoughtful evaluation for metabolic disorders is important in children with autism to determine possible metabolic dysfunctions and to guide treatments.

▶ C. THE IMMUNE SYSTEM

The immune system of the body is intricate. In addition to defending against infections, there is a complex intercommunication among immune cells and with other organ systems, including the brain.

The goals of the immune system are to:
1. Recognize potential harm from invaders (e.g., infectious organisms)
2. Contain or eliminate the infection/invader
3. Regulate and control the immune response to avoid damage to the body
4. Remember exposures in order to be able to react more quickly and robustly with subsequent exposures

The immediate defenders of the body are the physical barriers of skin and mucous membranes. Once invaders make it past this first line of defense, various immune responses are triggered.

Problems with the immune system can be divided into categories:
1. Immune deficiency or dysfunction: a defective or ineffective response
2. Hypersensitivity: overreaction to innocuous foreign material, out of proportion to potential damage (as seen in allergic responses)
3. Imbalanced reactions: decreased response to potentially dangerous infections and overreaction to things that may not be harmful
4. Autoimmunity: an inappropriate reaction to one's own cells or tissues
5. Inflammation: too vigorous of an attack against invaders with "bystander" damage to normal tissue

Energy Metabolism

The Immune System

A child with autism may have any or all of these challenges, to a greater degree than children with ADHD or those without behavioral/developmental disorders. These problems underlie some of the clinical problems seen in autism and are amenable to treatment.

The immune system is like a complex military defense system with many divisions, subdivisions, and specialists working together. The basic divisions include white blood cells, antibodies, and chemical messengers called cytokines. Some of these cytokines promote inflammation while others help combat it. A balanced response is necessary to protect against invaders and then stop the reaction to prevent damage. A detailed discussion of the various types of immune cells and functions is beyond the scope of this book. Please see the resources listed in the references section for more information.

Immune Problems in Children with ADHD and Autism

The following problems are primarily seen in a subset of children with autism. Children with ADHD may have allergies but do not typically have the immune system deficiencies or dysfunctions that may be seen in autism.

Immune deficiency. Many studies show that children with autism have low to normal immunoglobulins (antibodies), low numbers of certain types of white blood cells (T cells), and/or low or poorly functioning natural killer cells (cells that kill viruses and other invaders). Some children have low secretory IgA, the antibody present in the lining of the GI and respiratory tracts, predisposing them to infections. Supplements that help improve secretory IgA include *Saccharomyces boulardii* (a beneficial yeast), probiotics, glutamine, omega-3 fatty acids, vitamin A, and zinc.

Hypersensitivity (allergies). The histamine chemical released in an allergy reaction can cause physical and behavioral symptoms. See section 2.1 Allergies for more information.

Imbalanced immune reactions. The following imbalanced reactions can be seen in a subset of children with autism:
1. Imbalanced Th1 and Th2 cells (specific subtypes of white blood cells)
2. Imbalanced cytokines (chemical messengers) with more cytokines that promote inflammation
3. Decreased or poor function of natural killer cells

These imbalanced reactions may also predispose children with autism to developing low-grade or subclinical (hard to recognize) viral infections, which may trigger inflammation.

Autoimmunity

In autoimmunity, the body inappropriately reacts to its own cells as if they were foreign invaders. Many types of autoantibodies have been found in children with autism. The significance of the many types of antibrain antibodies (e.g., antimyelin antibodies, etc.) is being actively investigated.

A subset of children with ADHD or autism can have a syndrome known as PANDAS (**P**ediatric **A**utoimmune **N**europsychiatric **D**isorders **A**ssociated with

Strep). Strep infection appropriately triggers the production of antibodies to fight off the infection. These antibodies then inappropriately react against a portion of the brain known as the basal ganglia, which results in increased obsessive–compulsive disorder (OCD) symptoms. PANDAS has recently been expanded to PANS (**P**ediatric **A**cute-onset **N**europsychiatric **S**yndrome), which can be induced by a broader range of microbes. Key features include acute and sudden onset of (or worsening of preexisting) OCD behaviors, tics, or other symptoms. Children with autism may also experience sudden overall behavioral regression.

A more recently described condition is cerebral folate deficiency, which is deficiency of the B vitamin folate in the spinal fluid. This can result in a variety of developmental disorders including autism. Antibodies are inappropriately made against the receptors that help transport folate into the spinal fluid. Treatment involves providing high doses of an easily utilizable form of folate called folinic acid along with decreasing triggers of these interfering antibodies. A casein-free diet is associated with lower levels of these problematic antibodies.

Inflammation
Inflammation can be an outcome of a dysfunctional immune system. A subset of children with autism have immune responses that do not turn off normally, staying activated or turned on and resulting in inflammation. Some children with autism have inflammatory bowel disease. Autopsy studies have reported low-grade chronic inflammation in the brains of children with autism. Inflammation is further described in Section 3.2 D: Inflammation.

Potential treatments for immune system problems include:
- Probiotics, which can modulate abnormal intestinal immune responses
- Treating triggers of inflammation such as allergies, intestinal bacterial imbalance, yeast overgrowth, and toxins
- Nutritional supplementation, such as glutamine; probiotics; *Saccharomyces boulardii*; vitamins A, D, and C; zinc; omega-3 fatty acids; quercetin; and curcumin

Continued investigation into the intricacies of the immune system and how it affects brain health and function will hopefully lead to more specific and effective treatments.

▶ D. THE NEUROLOGIC SYSTEM

Since ADHD and autism are considered "brain disorders," it would seem logical that the source of the problem is primarily in the brain. There are certainly primary brain conditions, both anatomic and functional, that affect brain function. There are genetic syndromes that include altered brain anatomy or function. Children with autism may have differences from other children such as in total brain size, size of different brain regions, and communication between areas of the brain.

The Neurologic System

However, in a newer paradigm of thinking, the brain may also be secondarily affected by issues outside of it. Rather than being static, fixed deficits that are permanent and not amenable to treatment, many seemingly brain-based symptoms may, in fact, have their origins outside of the brain. In addition, brain "plasticity," the ability of the brain to alter its biological, chemical, and physical properties in reaction to physiological stressors, was long thought to be a process that was only present during a critical period in early childhood. More recent studies show that brain plasticity occurs throughout life.

In this newer model, there are many potential contributing factors to poor brain function.

- Nutrient deficiencies, such as in precursors for neurotransmitters (e.g., tryptophan for serotonin) and other important nutrients for brain structure, development, and function (e.g., DHA)
- Elevated histamine from allergies
- Food intolerances and sensitivities, including opiate-like reactions
- Toxins from:
  - Inadequate elimination of the body's own metabolic toxic by-products
  - Imbalanced or excessive intestinal bacteria (including *Clostridia*) and/or yeast
  - External toxin sources
- Inflammation
- Imbalance of excitatory and inhibitory (calming) transmitters

These abnormalities can be seen in children with ADHD or autism. Individuals with autism have many more potential contributing factors to brain dysfunction than individuals with ADHD, which may in part explain the difference in depth, breadth, and severity of symptoms between the two disorders.

Neurological Problems in Children with ADHD and Autism

Secondary effects on brain function that are discussed elsewhere include:
- Food sensitivities and intolerances (GI discussion earlier in this section and section 4.17 Digestive Enzymes)
- Toxins from yeast or problematic bacteria (section 2.18 Yeast Overgrowth)
- Histamine from allergies (section 2.1 Allergies)

These functional problems can only occur if problematic substances are able to enter the brain. This requires an understanding of the blood–brain barrier.

Blood–Brain Barrier

The brain has a built-in protective barrier, the blood–brain barrier, which lets helpful substances in and keeps potentially harmful substances out. The blood–brain barrier separates blood from brain tissue and the fluid in the brain. Unfortunately, this barrier can be compromised by a number of factors including high blood pressure, infection, inflammation, ischemia (inadequate blood flow and oxygen), injury/trauma, and immune challenges to the barrier itself.

There are also regions around the base of the brain that are intentionally more permeable so that they can sense the external environment and chemical state of the blood and respond appropriately. Toxins can also potentially enter the brain through these permeable areas.

Brain Cells: Neurons and Glial Cells

To further understand some of what can go wrong in the brain, especially in children with autism, it is first necessary to review the various types of cells in the brain and their functions.

Commonly discussed are neurons, the cells that send messages from one nerve cell to another across spaces called synapses. Messages are sent via neurotransmitters, which are chemicals released from a nerve cell to transmit an impulse from one nerve cell to another.

Less discussed but vitally important are glial cells, or glia. Glia means "glue," and these cells were initially thought to be unimportant cells holding the rest of the brain together. We now know that they are active and extremely important for brain functioning. Glial cells make up the bulk of the brain and provide different and interconnected functions based on three types:

- Microglia, which protect the brain cells, send out inflammatory cytokines (chemical messengers) causing oxidative stress (creation of substances called free radicals, which can potentially damage cell walls and DNA) and inflammation, and get rid of pathogens and cellular debris
- Oligodendrocytes, which coat axons (connector neurons) with a protective sheath called myelin, and are highly susceptible to oxidative stress
- Astrocytes, which make up the bulk of glial cells, form part of the blood–brain barrier, anchor neurons to their blood supply, process sensory information, supply nutrients and glutathione to neurons, get rid of excitotoxic glutamate, and clean up brain debris and toxins

The excess glutamate and insufficient GABA imbalance that can result when astrocytes are overwhelmed by toxins and other insults is an important contributing factor to brain dysfunction in autism.

Potential Problems in the Brains of Children with Autism

Glia also have a role in the regulation of repair of neurons after injury. When any or all of these processes are overwhelmed, damaged, or poorly regulated, problems can develop.

The good news is that glial cells can regenerate, and infectious and inflammatory triggers can be identified and treated. Nutrients and cofactor supplements can decrease oxidative stress and help restore a more ideal excitatory-inhibitory balance. This makes the previously described scenario amenable to treatment.

For more information and exquisite descriptions of this process, refer to the book *The Autism Revolution* by Martha Herbert, M.D., Ph.D.

Additional problems include:

Toxins. These can come from many sources, including external sources, such as heavy metals (see section 5.1 Toxic Metals); the GI tract, such as toxins

The Neurologic System

produced as a result of bacteria and yeast overgrowth in the intestine; and impaired elimination of toxins from normal cellular metabolism.

The chemical glutathione is critical in the body's ability to detoxify. Glutathione is an antioxidant with protective effects in the brain. A significant number of children with autism have deficiencies in glutathione, predisposing them to more adverse effects from toxin exposure (see the section on sulfation page 166).

Neuroinflammation. Autopsy studies have documented chronic low-grade inflammation in the brains of children with autism. Inflammation is a consequence of the disordered processes described above and can interfere with brain health and functioning. This is a potentially treatable condition, by eliminating or minimizing triggers of inflammation and providing anti-inflammatory nutrients.

Seizures. The question of seizures often arises in children with ADHD and inattention symptoms. The vast majority of staring episodes in ADHD are *not* seizures. Consider seizures when a child has frequent staring episodes, does not respond when his or her name is called (not simply due to overfocusing), or the episodes are accompanied by lip smacking, eye movements, or hand/finger movements.

Individuals with autism have a higher incidence of seizures (up to 35 percent) than typically developing children (1 to 2 percent). Consider a neurological evaluation and EEG (recording of brain wave activity) for seizures if your child has unexplained developmental or language regression or frequent or prolonged staring episodes and is unresponsive to interaction. There are nutrients that may be helpful for seizures, but these should only be considered after appropriate medical evaluation and in coordination with a child's treating physician.

Additional findings suggest brain changes in autism may not be "fixed," (i.e., permanent). For example, fever can improve function and behavior, reducing "autistic" symptoms, in a subset of children with autism. The exact cause of this improvement is not yet known. Improved behavior during fever is *not* consistent with a permanent, untreatable brain condition. Exposures to some triggers of inflammation can result in prolonged increases in certain pro-inflammatory chemicals (cytokines) in the brain; this can mimic a more permanent, static brain condition.

Potential Treatments

Given an understanding of the above problems, potential treatments to help overall brain function can therefore include:

- Correcting nutritional deficiencies and providing nutrients needed to make brain transmitters
- Eliminating triggers for inflammation and providing anti-inflammatory supplements
- Treating traditional allergies and lowering histamine
- Restoring intestinal health and balance

- Eliminating problematic foods
- Eliminating sources of toxins and supporting the body's own detoxification processes
- Restoring appropriate balance between excitatory and inhibitory transmitters in the brain

Nutrients important in brain structure, development and function include:
- Omega-3 fatty acids, especially DHA
- Magnesium
- Zinc
- Copper
- B vitamins, especially B_{12}, folinic acid, B_6, and B_3 (niacinamide)
- TMG
- Vitamin C
- Amino acid precursors to neurotransmitters (e.g., tryptophan, tyrosine, choline, glutamine, GABA)

■ 3.2 Barriers and Bottlenecks: The Four Primary Mechanisms

▶ A. METHYLATION
By Elizabeth Mumper, M.D., F.A.A.P., President and CEO of the Rimland Center

Every second in every cell in every organ of every human, there are exquisitely orchestrated biochemical reactions working in sequence to make neurotransmitters, proteins, and cell membranes. Think of biochemistry as a sequence of interlocking gears. When all the appropriate enzymes and catalysts are present and functioning properly, the gears turn smoothly. When there is a weakness in an enzyme or a catalyst malfunctions, one of the gears locks up. Methylation biochemistry is fundamental to human life, yet quite complex to understand.

Methylation is a critical process in human metabolism because it takes care of your DNA and RNA. The process turns gene expression off or on depending upon the situation, the tissue involved, and what the body needs. Methylation helps in the development of neurotransmitters including dopamine, which is involved in cognition, mood, behavior, attention, and learning. Many medications marketed for ADHD are designed to increase dopamine levels. Methylation also helps build flexible cell membranes, which allow for the entry of substances such as minerals, medications, and mood-enhancing neurotransmitters as well as the removal of toxins. Methylation also makes creatine for energy.

Methylation is the act of attaching a methyl group (a carbon atom and three hydrogen atoms) to another substance. Then transsulfuration begins with the production of homocysteine (from methylation) and makes glutathione, which is important for lots of reasons for children with ADHD or autism.

Methylation is one way you turn your genes off and on. Genes are proteins. When a methyl group is attached, the gene is silenced; when a methyl group leaves, the gene is activated. Imagine a gene that controls cell growth. If you are a baby, it is important to have that gene unmethylated, therefore expressed, so that you can grow and develop. If you are an adult with cancer, you might wish for that gene to be methylated (silenced) so that your tumor does not grow.

Two biochemical cycles, or "gears," make methyl groups available. One gear is the methylation cycle. As the methylation cycle gear turns, methionine is converted to S-adenosyl-methionine, nature's go-to methyl donor. Further biochemical reactions generate homocysteine, which is re-methylated back to make more methionine in a perfect example of recycling, or undergoes further conversions to make glutathione in a stellar example of multitasking.

Another gear is the folate cycle. As the folate cycle gear turns, an inactive form of folate is converted to an active form; in the process a methyl group is made available to contribute to the methylation cycle. Folate is crucial for several reasons: making proteins, helping the nervous system, and scavenging free radicals.

So when the methylation cycle is functioning like a smoothly turning gear, you go about your day while your cellular biochemistry makes fatty, juicy cell membranes, keeps your neurotransmitters such as dopamine in good supply, and turns thousands of genes off and on depending on the organs they are in and the jobs they need to do.

Meanwhile, another cycle (sulfation) includes glorious glutathione, which was synthesized from homocysteine and is busy with a diverse repertoire of functions: acting as the body's primary intracellular antioxidant, serving as the gateway to detoxification biochemistry, repairing the lining of the gut, supporting mitochondrial function, and helping the T cells of the immune system.

Visualize these three gears turning smoothly and in concert with one another. Now imagine what kinds of things could go wrong to disrupt the whole process. The analogy of biochemistry to mechanics is imperfect and simplified. Biochemical gear turning depends upon a series of reactions in which one substance is converted to another substance. In turn, those reactions are typically dependent on enzymes, which require minerals or nutrients that facilitate the reactions. Deficiencies that disrupt enzyme function can therefore cause problems. For example, if a child is born with a weakness in one of the enzymes needed for a biochemical conversion, the gear could get stuck. If the child is low in a specific nutrient or mineral, the gears might not rotate as well.

Vitamins including folinic acid, B_{12} in the methylated form (methylcobalamin), pyridoxyl-5′-phosphate (an active form of B_6), and minerals such as zinc and magnesium keep these three biochemical gears functioning smoothly and working together. In an ideal world, children would get their nutrition from food. This is not the case for some children with autism and ADHD, who require higher levels of targeted nutritional supplementation, based on an analysis of biomarkers that can help the clinician determine which part of these crucial cycles is not functioning well. This determination can lead to gratifying clinical improvements.

▶ B. SULFATION

There is an intimate relationship between methylation and sulfation. If methylation stalls out, sulfation does too. Sulfur from dietary sources and amino acids are critical in human health. Sulfation is the addition of sulfur to another molecule. Sulfation is involved in immune cell infection-fighting ability; producing energy from the mitochondria (generator); neurotransmitter breakdown; preventing oxidation (rusting) of the cells; and ridding the body of toxins. The liver uses sulfate to change toxins into forms that can be eliminated.

Sulfation depletion occurs when there is inadequate sulfate in the diet or a lack of the nutrients necessary for methylation, sulfation, and coping with oxidative stress. The toxic load level also makes a difference, depending upon each individual's detoxification capacity. Like straws on the camel's back, outcome depends upon the strength of the camel and the total load.

Toxin Challenges to Sulfation

From our own metabolism, toxic by-products are produced that need to be handled and removed—like taking out the garbage. Some individuals have faulty "disposal" systems that allow their "garbage" metabolites to build up in the body and recycle, increasing the demand on toxin removal even more. There are also external sources: foods laden with artificial additives and preservatives, water contaminated with chemicals, and air abundant with industrial chemicals and pollutants. We have manufactured (human-made) chemicals everywhere—in our clothing, personal care products, food containers, cookware, and lawn care and pest control treatments. According to the EPA, there are approximately 84,000 synthetic chemicals in the environment. These were not present until approximately the last 200 years, and only 200 have been tested.

These toxins are ubiquitous and here to stay, with potentially tragic effects on developing fetuses, infants, and children. In addition to avoiding toxic exposures to the extent possible, we must provide children with the raw materials to improve their detoxification capabilities.

Detoxification "Disposals" in the Cells

There are a number of systems in the body for metabolizing organic compounds and also ridding our "garbage" from internal metabolism and external sources. The main set of systems is similar to a dual-phase disposal: phase I (cytochrome P450s) and phase II (glucuronidation and sulfation).

Another sulfation system involves phenol sulfotransferase (PST) enzymes for metabolizing phenols abundant in healthy foods, but excessive in artificial additives, coloring, and salicylate-containing medications. The total phenol intake, in sensitive individuals, can exceed the supply of available sulfate. (See section 2.15 Silly Behavior for symptoms of phenol reactions and treatments.) Glutathione in the final sulfation stage is known as "the garbage bag" of detox. The body must be hardy to keep the supply of glutathione "garbage bags" adequate to meet the usual demands of metabolism as well as those from the diet and toxic environment.

Sulfation

Although all of us are exposed to these toxins, the ability to detox efficiently lies in the exposure level (load) relative to the individual's "disposal" capacity. Many individuals have detoxification inefficiencies that render them vulnerable to what may be "insignificant" toxin exposures to others.

The body cannot produce sulfate on its own, and depends upon dietary intake from proteins, cruciferous vegetables (broccoli, cauliflower, and brussels sprouts), legumes, onions, and garlic. Other nutrients that support sulfation and glutathione metabolism include sulfur amino acids (methionine, cysteine, taurine, N-acetyl cysteine), magnesium, alpha-lipoic acid, selenium, copper, zinc, and vitamins B_2 and B_3. Magnesium sulfate via Epsom salts baths and/or topical lotion is effective in providing the needed sulfate. (See section 2.10 Hyperactivity—section D).

The collaborative team of methylation and sulfation provides the backbone for the body's core functions. Understanding the pair leads us naturally to the next section on the challenges of oxidative stress.

▶ C. OXIDATION

In our analogy of the gears, methylation and sulfation, think of oxidation as the rust in the gears. It causes damage. Oxidation is a necessary process in the body where oxygen combines with another substance to produce an oxide. When there is a disease challenge, the body can convert a small amount of the oxygen into free radicals that are the bullets fired to get rid of disease-causing agents. However, this process can spin out of control and consequently, the excess free-radical "bullets" cause collateral damage to the body tissues. The problems result from an excess chain reaction that may also trigger inflammation. This problem escalates until something halts it. The free radical, if not neutralized, can damage cell walls or DNA.

Enter the antioxidant nutrients that are taken in and antioxidant enzymes produced by the body to quench the oxidant attacks and stop the collateral damage. Antioxidant nutrients include vitamin C, vitamin E, vitamin A, selenium, zinc, coenzyme Q_{10}, glutathione, taurine, alpha-lipoic acid, cysteine, and more. Some plant substances with antioxidant functions include carotenoids, flavonoids, catechins, resveratrol, quercetin, proanthocyanidins, and isoflavones. High-antioxidant spices include cinnamon, oregano, and cloves. Foods high in antioxidants are fruits and vegetables, particularly garlic, onions, shallots, blueberries, guava, cruciferous vegetables, and some legumes, nuts, and seeds.

The free-radical process is worsened by our exposure to external sources of natural and synthetic environmental toxins and chemicals. While our planet's inhabitants have always been exposed to natural toxins (toxic metals, poisonous insects, snakes, and plants, etc.), it is only recently that we have experienced the additional burden of 84,000 human-made chemicals and ionizing radiation. Dietary sources of antioxidants are insufficient to compensate for the burden of oxidative stress.

The Methylation/Sulfation/Oxidative Stress Connection to Autism
There are documented differences in the biochemistry of children with autism that make them more vulnerable to oxidative stress. Jill James, Ph.D., a preeminent researcher in this field, has reported the following findings in children with autism, compared to controls:

- Lower DNA methylation (hypomethylation), which affects gene expression
- Decreased ratio of SAM (a methyl donor) to SAH (the methylation by-product), which is an indicator of reduced (poor) methylation capacity
- Increased biomarkers for oxidative stress

We are rapidly using up our precious reserves and maxing out our methylation, sulfation, and antioxidant defenses. It is not a surprise that the most vulnerable among us (developing fetuses, infants, and children) are paying the price for the industrial revolution that accelerated in the 1950s with the slogan "better living through chemistry." What we can and must do is identify those at risk and provide them with the preventive and therapeutic measures necessary to restore health and function.

▶ D. INFLAMMATION
Inflammation is a factor underlying many diseases in our society today, including acute and most chronic diseases, as well ADHD and autism. Inflammation is the body's normal response to injury or infection, calling in the cells the body needs to address the acute problem. When inflammation is directed at a perceived insult and short term, it is appropriate. When the reaction is excessive or does not turn off, inflammation can then become chronic, which leads to a variety of problems. As discussed previously, individuals with autism have many differences in their immune system that tend to favor the development of inflammation. The main organ systems affected by inflammation in children with autism, and to a lesser degree in children with ADHD, are the intestine and the brain.

Intestinal Inflammation
Intestinal inflammation commonly occurs in response to imbalances in the organisms that live there. When this balance of intestinal bacteria is disrupted, other organisms such as yeast or problematic bacteria can flourish, leading to local inflammation. Treatments involve restoring appropriate balance of the beneficial bacteria and eliminating excess yeast or problematic bacteria or parasites. Other sources of intestinal inflammation may include food reactions, toxic exposures, infectious agents, and/or the effects of medications

A subset of children with autism may also have inflammatory bowel disease, with findings similar to Crohn's disease or ulcerative colitis. Inflammation of this degree generally requires the involvement of a GI specialist and use of traditional medications.

Oxidation

Inflammation

Brain Inflammation

Important research from Johns Hopkins University in 2005 involved autopsy studies of the brains from eleven individuals with autism, ranging in age from five to forty-four years. They found widespread activation of inflammatory cells (microglia and astrocytes) in the individuals' brains.

The findings are relevant to autism because both microglia and astroglia are essential for nerve transmission function and brain development. Although the reaction is considered innate, it is certainly possible that stress from external sources (poor diet/nutrition, toxins, infections, etc.) can have a secondary negative effect on the health and function of the brain by limiting the exposure to needed nutrients. Simply, if the demands on the brain exceed the ability of the microglia and astrocytes to handle these demands, there can be problems in the brain including inflammation. For an exquisite description of brain mechanisms and potential treatments, refer to the book *The Autism Revolution* by Martha Herbert, M.D., Ph.D..

■ 3.3 *Stop Signs and Green Lights: Epigenetics— How Environment Affects Genes*

The *epi* portion of the term epigenetics is Greek for "over, above, or outer." Epigenetics is what surrounds the genes. In the past, it was thought that, with the exception of rare mutations (damage), genes were stable and not subject to change. The standard thinking was that DNA provided the instructions to make RNA, and RNA created proteins that control all cell activity. It is not that simple.

With the discovery of epigenetics, we now have a greater understanding of how environment profoundly influences genes by turning them on or off, changing how genes express themselves. The effect can be beneficial or not depending upon the individual's genetics and innate "programming" as influenced by the positives and negatives in the environment. The changes in the gene programming affect not only the individual but future generations.

According to Jill James, Ph.D., "Primary epigenetic mechanisms are DNA methylation and histone modifications (amino acid methylation/acetylation). By analogy, if genetic sequence is the hard drive, epigenetics is the software that determines whether, how, and when the sequence will be read."

Gene variants, different forms of genes that vary according to their DNA sequencing, also need to be considered. Gene variants may or may not be damaging. They are heritable and can be passed on. There are specific maternal and fetal gene variants that have been identified as increasing risk for autism.

The best example of epigenetics lies in identical twins. They possess the same genes, yet twins may have different illnesses and outcomes, particularly as they age and live in differing environments. If there is a predisposition to diabetes and one twin takes a proactive preventive diet and lifestyle approach and the other twin does the opposite, the outcomes will be proportionally different. Nonhereditary lifestyle factors influenced the gene expression to be beneficial in one twin and detrimental to the other.

Another compelling example, depicted in the *National Geographic* issue on twins (January 2012), describes identical twins, both of whom have autism, but with different presentations. Sam has Asperger's syndrome and is high functioning, while John has severe autism. Sam's first six months were healthy. Conversely, John's had multiple surgeries, with numerous exposures to anesthesia and strong medications. Their environment after birth likely changed the trajectory of their common predisposition to autism. In the Stanford Study of 192 twin pairs and autism, genes were found to have a 38 percent influence on the development of autism as compared to the environmental influence of 62 percent *(Hallmayer et al. Arch Gen Psychiatry. July 4, 2011).*

As described in the previous section on faulty mechanisms, many individuals with autism have dysfunctions in the methylation pathway. One of the important functions of methylation is gene expression—turning genes on and off.

What Does the Environment Include?

The environment includes lifestyle positives and negatives: what we eat and drink, the air we breathe, how we live our lives, and our exposures. The exposures can include toxins, pollutants, radiation, medications, vaccinations, nutritional supplements, products we use, and exercise.

For the developing fetus, the "womb environment" profoundly influences the future of that child. Human studies have revealed that a mother with a gene variant that impairs her methylation ability is more likely to have a child with autism or other developmental delays. Prenatal maternal exposures that can increase the risk for autism and developmental delays in the child include alcohol, infections, medications, toxins, fevers, and more.

The purpose of epigenetics is to regulate the processes in the body. According to Dr. Jean-Pierre Issa at the M.D. Anderson Cancer Center in a PBS interview, only 10 to 20 percent of genes are active in any cell. This prevents genes of one cell type from being expressed in another. For example, the gene for eye color only expresses in the eyes, not the liver, skin, or brain. In times of drought (an environmental challenge), the body produces molecules to modify DNA and turn on or off genes that help it endure difficult circumstances. These modifications affect many generations.

Appreciating the significance of epigenetics expands the treatment potential for a multiplicity of disorders, including autism and ADHD. We are already utilizing the findings that parents and their children with autism may share similar metabolic deficits in methylation and glutathione-dependent antioxidant and detoxification capacity. Scientific studies validate our own observations that maternal preconception and prenatal vitamin supplementation can reduce the risk for autism in the child, even when the mother and/or child have gene variants associated with increased risk for autism. The research has provided the science that enables us to identify these deficits and treat responsibly with the appropriate nutritional interventions.

Epigenetics

Tuning the Engine: Nutrients and Their Impact on Impaired Systems and Out-of-Sync Mechanisms

This chapter provides expanded information on vitamins, minerals, amino acids, carnitine, coenzyme Q_{10}, essential fatty acids, probiotics, and digestive enzymes. In addition to describing functions, risk for deficiencies, deficiency disorders, and deficiency signs and symptoms, we discuss the ADHD and autism connections along with supplementation specifics including products and goal dosing.

A chart in each section includes possible side effects, toxicity, food sources, and interactions. Within the interactions, we use specific terms to describe the effect of the individual's conditions, and impact of other nutrients, medications, toxins, and/or herbs on the presented nutrient's availability for use, digestion, absorption, transport, bioavailability, and/or function.
- Enhancers: benefit the nutrient of focus
- Antagonists: impede, deplete, or interfere with the nutrient of focus
- Competitors: compete with the nutrient of focus

VITAMINS
■ 4.1 Vitamin A and Beta-Carotene
Vitamin A and beta-carotene are both called vitamin A; however, they are distinctly different in their structures, absorption, effectiveness, functions, storage, toxicity, and sources.

Retinol is preformed vitamin A which is stored as retinyl esters in animal source foods (liver, fish, meat, and milk products). Absorption is enhanced by fat and is highest when tissue status is deficient. Vitamin A is stored primarily in the liver. As a fat-soluble vitamin, it can be toxic (unlike beta-carotene).

Preformed vitamin A is the most effective form of vitamin A. For most functions, beta-carotene needs to convert to vitamin A. Vitamin A retinoids also have many more functions than beta-carotene.

Provitamin A carotenoids, especially beta-carotene, are compounds that are precursors to vitamin A. Beta-carotene is found primarily in plant foods (orange/yellow vegetables and fruits) and also in egg yolks. Absorption improves with juicing and cooking.

Beta-carotene is stored in the fat cells, liver, and retina. It consists of two molecules of retinal that are cleaved in the intestines via a vitamin E–dependent step, then converted in the liver to retinol (vitamin A). Conversion efficiency is poor and some individuals do not convert well. Beta-carotene is nontoxic.

COMPARISON OF PREFORMED VITAMIN A AND BETA-CAROTENE

	VITAMIN A RETINOL—PREFORMED A	BETA-CAROTENE PROVITAMIN A
Functions	Epithelial integrity Growth Immunity Cell differentiation Retina structure and function Cornea structure and function Reproduction Anticancer: breast, bladder, cervical Stored in liver	Antioxidant Respiratory epithelial function

Risks for deficiency	Poor absorption
	Celiac disease
	Low-fat diet
	Low-protein diet
	Diarrhea
	Alcohol
	Diseases: liver, pancreas, kidney
	Laxative use
	Cystic fibrosis
	Parasites
		Poor absorption
		Celiac disease
		Poor conversion in:
		  Diabetes
		  Hypothyroidism
		Alcohol
		Caffeine
		Laxatives

Deficiency disorders	Xerophthalmia (dry ridged conjunctiva and cornea)
	Bitot's spots (rough gray deposits on conjunctiva)
	Blindness
	Keratomalacia (ulceration of cornea)
	Hyperkeratosis (thickening of the cornea)
	Fetus birth defects:
	  Cleft palate
	  Vision impairment to blindness
	  Keratomalacia
		See vitamin A

Deficiency symptoms	Vision dysfunctions Night blindness Abnormal cornea Immune dysfunction Increased infections Acne Eczema Dry skin and eyes Dermatitis Lichen planus Keratosis pilaris ("chicken skin") Ridged nails Hypothyroidism	Excess free radicals Poor lung epithelium Aching joints Low T cells Visual disturbances

Vitamin A Supplements

Preformed vitamin A is the most efficient and well-utilized form of A and is preferred over beta-carotene. Vitamin A (preformed) types:

- Retinoids (retinol, retinal, and retinoic acids) are found only in animal and fish products.
  - Most naturally occurring retinoids are in the retinyl palmitate form.
  - If the vitamin A is from natural sources, the label will indicate vitamin A from fish oils.
- Micellized vitamin A is a water-soluble form of vitamin A, which is less toxic and well absorbed, especially in malabsorption conditions such as celiac disease. In the intestines, micelle formation occurs in via bile salts allowing absorption of lipids and fat-soluble vitamins. Micellized forms bypass this step and are more easily absorbed.
- Synthetic vitamin A palmitate is derived from vitamin A acetate, a synthetic organic chemical. This form is commonly used in commercial dairy products and other commercial foods. If the label states "vitamin A palmitate," it may be natural or synthetic. Vitamin A from fish oil sources is preferred.

Vitamin A and the Connection to ADHD and Autism

Vitamin A deficiency has been noted in a subset of children with autism and is not prevalent in ADHD. Zinc deficiency is also common in autism. The retinol-binding protein that transports vitamin A for utilization is zinc dependent. The more profound the zinc deficiency, the greater the negative impact on vitamin A function.

Eye contact. Vitamin A (not beta-carotene) is critical for vision, especially night vision. When the retina of the eye is deprived of vitamin A, rod and cone function are impaired. While we do not fully understand how vitamin A affects eye contact, the clinical experience is impressive. When vitamin A deficiency is a significant factor, improvements in eye contact may be seen within weeks of adequate supplementation. Sideways glancing declines or resolves and the child makes direct eye contact without prompting.

Skin problems: eczema and dermatitis. The most common cause of vitamin A deficiency is zinc deficiency, which is why they share some of the same symptoms. Vitamin A is necessary for the maintenance and repair of external and internal epithelial tissues. Deficiency can result in epithelial inflammation, eczema, dermatitis, acne, and the classical vitamin A deficiency symptom, keratosis pilaris ("chicken skin" bumps on arms and thighs). Mucosal epithelial tissues are also affected, increasing the risk for gingivitis, rhinitis, sinusitis, gastritis, colitis, and more.

Immunity and inflammation. Immune dysfunctions and the presence of inflammation are common in autism but not in ADHD. Vitamin A has a broad effect on white blood cell functions, histamine, healing, repair, and many immune mediators in the body.

VITAMIN A TOTAL DAILY GOAL DOSING

AGE	DAILY DOSE
2 to 3	1,250 IU
4 to 5	1,250 to 2,500 IU
6 to 10	2,500 to 3,500 IU
11 +	3,500 to 5,000 IU

- Account for all sources of preformed vitamin A.
- If taking a multivitamin while also taking either cod liver oil or a separate vitamin A supplement, use a vitamin that does not contain preformed vitamin A.
- Many forms of cod liver oil have variable amounts of vitamin A per serving size, some with a very wide range (e.g., from 0 to 1,500 IU/serving). Use a cod liver oil that provides a consistent amount of vitamin A per serving.
- If using cod liver oil in liquid form, the supplement will also provide omega-3 fatty acids (EPA and DHA). However, cod liver oil soft gels primarily provide vitamins A and D and not much essential fatty acids.
- Many commercially available micellized vitamin A drops are too high in concentration for use in younger children; compounding of a lower dose drop may be necessary.
- Beta-carotene may be taken along with vitamin A, because carotenoids only convert to vitamin A when body stores are inadequate. Therefore, carotenoids do not result in vitamin A toxicity.

Zinc intake must be adequate. Zinc is critical for retinol-binding protein, which is essential for vitamin A transport. Zinc converts retinol to retinal, the form of vitamin A necessary for rod cell function, which is responsible for night vision and dark adaptation.

Zinc supplements
- Well tolerated: gluconates, chelates, citrates, acetates, picolinates, chlorides, and bisglycinates
- Strong taste, needs disguising: sulfates

ZINC TOTAL DAILY GOAL DOSING

AGE	DOSE	FREQUENCY	TOTAL DAILY DOSE FROM ALL SOURCES
2 to 5	5 to 10 mg	1 or 2 times per day	10 to 20 mg
6 to 10	10 mg	2 times per day	20 mg
11 +	10 to 15 mg	2 times per day	20 to 30 mg

See section 4.9 Zinc for more information.

Vitamin D intake must be adequate. Excess intakes of vitamin A or vitamin D are antagonistic to the other. It is important to include vitamin D whenever vitamin A supplementation is recommended and vice versa. See the section 4.2 Vitamin D.

VITAMIN A AND BETA-CAROTENE

	VITAMIN A RETINOL—PREFORMED A	BETA-CAROTENE PROVITAMIN A
Diagnostic tests	Serum vitamin A Retinol-binding protein (serum) Dark adaptation	Serum beta-carotene
Supplement types	Vitamin A from fish oil sources Fish oils containing vitamin A Micellized A for better absorption	Beta-carotenoid is the most efficient precursor to vitamin A compared to other carotenoids
Possible side effects	Irritability	Skin tone slightly yellow/orange
Toxicity	>30,000 IU long term	None. When body stores are sufficient, beta-carotene will not convert to vitamin A
Excess/toxicity side effects	Headache Scaly skin Bone loss Double vision Low vitamin D Birth defects: eyes, head, face	Deep yellow/orange color to skin from tissue retention of the carotenoids Does not cause vitamin A toxicity
Sources	Retinyl palmitate found in animal sources: beef liver, milk products, fish and fish liver oils	Yellow/orange vegetables and fruits Egg yolks
Interactions	*Beneficial:* fat, bile, vitamin E, zinc, protein *Competitor:* high dose vitamin D	*Enhancers:* bile, fatty acids, vitamins E and C, zinc, thyroid

■ *4.2 Vitamin D*

Vitamin D is a fat-soluble vitamin that serves many important functions. It is found in some foods, is added to others, and is available as a supplement. It also comes from exposure to sunlight, which triggers the conversion of cholesterol in the skin to vitamin D. Vitamin D is important for strong, healthy bones and for many other aspects of overall health.

Functions

- Calcium absorption
- Bone growth and remodeling
- Tooth development
- Collagen
- Anti-inflammatory
- Immune support
- Brain development
- Neurotransmitter support
- Neuromuscular function
- Modulation of cell growth
- Decreased cancer risk

Risks for deficiency
- Inadequate dietary intake
- Poor digestion and/or absorption (especially impaired fat absorption)
- Limited sun exposure or individuals with darker skin tone
- Celiac disease
- Breastfeeding without vitamin D supplementation of the infant
- Excess vitamin A intake
- Medications (e.g., Phenobarbital, Dilantin, antacids, steroids, and laxatives)
- Vitamin D receptor defect

Deficiency disorders and associated conditions
- Rickets
- Osteomalacia
- Osteoporosis
- Low calcium and tetany (muscle spasm)
- Hypothyroidism
- Impaired fetal and child development
- Failure to thrive

Deficiency signs and symptoms
- Frontal bossing (prominent forehead)
- Bowlegged (from mild to severe)
- Rib bulges
- Profuse sweating
- Muscle or bone pain
- Delayed tooth eruption
- Scaly, cracked lips
- Eczema, dermatitis
- Seizures
- Seasonal affective disorder
- Delayed fontanelle closure (soft spot on scalp)
- Impaired cognitive function
- Communication delays
- Weight gain
- Increased risk for: diabetes, cardiovascular disease, specific cancers, autoimmunity, depression, and obesity

Vitamin D supplements
- Vitamin D_3 (cholecalciferol) is the best form to utilize for supplementation.
- Vitamin D_2 (ergocalciferol) converts to vitamin D_3 and is less effective long term.
- Vitamin D_3 is available in capsules, tablets, and liquids.
- The micellized version of vitamin D_3 is a water-soluble form of vitamin D that is well absorbed and especially useful in malabsorption conditions.
- The oil and micellized forms are preferred over the dry forms.

Vitamin D

VITAMIN D₃ SUPPLEMENTS

VITAMIN D₃ CHOLECALCIFEROL	AMOUNT	COMMENTS
Vitamin D drops, made by *Carlson, Nordic Naturals*	400 IU/drop	Easy to give
Vitamin D₃ capsules	400 IU/caps	There are capsules from 1,000 IU to 5,000 IU *Use these only under the care of a practitioner*
Micellized Vitamin D₃ drops, made by *Klaire Labs, Biotics Bio-D-Mulsion*	400 IU/drop	Biotics Bio-D-Mulsion is 2,000 IU drops *Use this only under the care of a practitioner*

VITAMIN D₃ IN COMBINATION WITH OMEGA-3 FATTY ACID SUPPLEMENTS

SUPPLEMENT COMPANY	DOSE	EPA	DHA	VITAMIN D₃	VITAMIN A	COMMENTS
ProOmega or Ultimate Omega with D₃, made by *Nordic Naturals*	½ tsp	813 mg	563 mg	500 IU	0	Lemon flavor
ProOmega or Ultimate Omega soft gels with D₃, made by *Nordic Naturals*	1 soft gel	650 mg	450 mg	500 IU	0	Lemon flavor in the soft gel
Baby's DHA (+ EPA), made by *Nordic Naturals*	4 ml	328 mg	480 mg	250 IU	340 to 1,200 IU	Well tolerated
Norwegian cod liver oil, made by *Carlson*	1 tsp	400 mg	500 mg	400 IU	850 IU	Lemon flavored
Cod liver oil with or without A and D₃, made by *Kirkman Labs*	½ tsp	250 mg	250 mg	250 IU	2,500 IU	Flavored (or unflavored)

Vitamin D and the Connection to ADHD and Autism

Vitamin D is a common deficiency in the general population and not necessarily unique to children with ADHD or autism. It is relevant to these disorders for its importance in physical and brain development, cognitive function, communication, mood, and behavior. Vitamin D (along with vitamin A, zinc, and omega-3 fatty acids) is important in skin health. In addition, its anti-inflammatory and immune-supporting functions are beneficial for children who have inflammation or immune issues, both of which are not uncommon in children with autism.

Vitamin D Supplements

- Dosing is dependent on blood level
- Minimum target blood level = 50 nmol/L
- For autism and/or anxiety, recommended level is 60 to 80 nmol/L

VITAMIN D TOTAL DAILY GOAL DOSING

AGE	DAILY DOSE
2 to 5	400 to 600 IU
6 to 10	600 to 800 IU
11 +	800 to 2,000 IU

- We recommend blood testing (25-hydroxy vitamin D).
- Higher doses may be required due to poor absorption or blood test results.
- Higher doses than recommended should be used under the guidance of a practitioner.

VITAMIN D (CHOLECALCIFEROL)

Tests	Serum 25-hydroxy vitamin D Acceptable range: 40 to 100 ng/mL Optimal level: 60 to 80 ng/mL
Possible side effects	None up to 10,000 IU
Toxicity	From supplements: unlikely at intakes of less than 10,000 IU per day. 50,000 IU daily long term has been demonstrated to be toxic. FNB recommends avoiding blood levels over 125 to 150 nmol/L. From sun exposure: None.
Toxic/excess side effects	Anorexia, weight loss, nausea, vomiting, constipation, weakness, excessive urination, bone pain, abnormal heart rhythms, and elevated calcium
Sources	Liver, fish oils, egg yolk, fatty fish, fortified milk, sunlight
Interactions	*Enhancers:* fat, bile *Antagonists*: corticosteroids (e.g., prednisone)—decreases vitamin D and calcium Antiseizure medications (e.g., phenobarbital, Dilantin)—metabolism of vitamin D to inactive compounds *Competitor.* high dose vitamin A

■ *4.3 Vitamin E (Tocopherol, Tocotrienol)*

Vitamin E is an essential nutrient occurring in four forms (alpha, beta, gamma, and delta tocopherols) and as tocotrienols. There is only a slight structural difference between tocotrienols and tocopherols. Tocotrienols occur in small amounts in specific vegetable oils, wheat germ, barley, saw palmetto, and specific grains and nuts.

Chemically, vitamin E in all of its forms functions as an antioxidant, protecting cell membranes, active enzyme sites, and DNA from free radical antioxidant damage (see section 3.2 Mechanisms: Oxidation). Tocotrienols are proving to be more effective in antioxidant capacity than tocopherols.

Vitamin E's protective functions also include immunity, lipids, muscles, nerves, and the brain.

Functions

- Antioxidant
- Maintains cell membrane integrity (by preventing lipid destruction)
- Protects from cardiovascular disease
- Protects fats in low-density lipo-proteins (LDLs) from oxidation by free radicals
- Protects against neurodegenerative disorders
- Transcription (process of transcrib-ing DNA information to RNA)
- Nerve function
- Muscle health
- Reproduction
- Anticlotting, by inhibiting platelet aggregation
- Cholesterol metabolism
- Expression and activities of immune and inflammatory cells
- Enhances dilation of blood vessels
- Life expectancy of red blood cells
- Fertility

Risks for deficiency

- Inadequate intake
- Severe malnutrition
- Fat malabsorption syndromes, including cystic fibrosis
- Hepatobiliary system disorders
- Genetic defects in the alpha-tocopherol transfer protein and/or in lipoproteins
- Medications that block fat absorption
- Laxatives
- Excess copper and iron
- Exposures to oxidative stress: pollutants, nitrous oxide, ozone, and pesticides

Deficiency disorders and associated conditions

- Abetalipoproteinemia (fat malab-sorption), which leads to Spinocer-ebellar ataxia (degenerative disease with poor coordination of gait and hand, speech and eye movements)
- Cholestatic liver disease
- Hemolytic anemia
- Myopathy (muscle damage)
- Pigmented retinopathy
- Hyperbilirubinemia (infant jaundice)

Deficiency signs and symptoms

- Absence of deep tendon reflexes
- Loss of vibratory sensation and proprioception
- Positive/abnormal Babinski sign (sign of brain disorder)
- Increased free radical damage to the red blood cells (RBC), resulting in anemia
- RBC fragility and reduced RBC life span
- Low HDL
- Sterility in males
- Miscarriage
- Hormonal disorders
- Retinal damage
- Cataracts

Vitamin E Supplements

The effective forms of both tocopherols and tocotrienols are the d forms (not the artificial l or dl forms). The Food and Nutrition Board has set recommendations on alpha-tocopherol only, not the other tocopherol forms, and no standards have been set on the trienols at this time.

Use of alpha-tocopherol forms alone is a concern because of interference with the use of other forms, particularly gamma-tocopherol. Although both alpha- and gamma-tocopherol are powerful antioxidants, gamma-tocopherol uniquely scavenges reactive nitrogen species that, like reactive oxygen species, are potent pro-oxidants and can damage proteins, lipids, and DNA. Gamma-tocopherol is also a better anti-inflammatory than the alpha form including its effects against neurodegenerative disorders.

For these reasons, we recommend a mixture of natural tocopherols over d-alpha-tocopherol only.

Vitamin E and the Connection to ADHD and Autism

Vitamin E is beneficial in any condition in which oxidation and inflammation are prevalent. These conditions are commonly seen in autism but may also be present in ADHD. Vitamin E, in combination with omega-3 fatty acids, has shown benefit in promoting speech in autism. Other roles include reducing excitotoxity noted in autism, and protection against neurodegeneration and muscle damage.

Vitamin E supplementation in autism and ADHD
- Mixed natural tocopherols
- Mixed natural tocopherols with tocotrienols

VITAMIN E TOTAL DAILY GOAL DOSING

AGE	DOSE	FREQUENCY
2 to 5	25 IU	Daily
6 to 10	50 IU	Daily
11 +	75 IU	Daily

Higher doses should be accomplished only under the guidance of a health care practitioner.

VITAMIN E (TOCOPHEROL)

Tests	Serum vitamin E (tocopherol) Tocopherol/triglyceride ratio (low = deficiency) Lipid peroxidation Red blood cell hemolysis Elevated bilirubin
Possible side effects	Easy bruising
Toxicity/excess side effects	More than 1,650 IU long term Severe bruising, easy bleeding GI distress Reduced carotene
Sources	Wheat germ, seeds, oils, eggs, grains, vegetables Amount available in food supply is limited

Vitamin E

VITAMIN E (TOCOPHEROL)—cont'd

Interactions	*Enhancers:* dietary fat, bile, selenium, vitamin C, beta-carotene *Antagonists:* cholestyramine, colestipol, isoniazid, mineral oil, orlistat, sucralfate, olestra *Increases risk of bleeding when taken with vitamin E:* anticoagulants, antiplatelet medications, NSAIDs

INTRODUCTION TO THE FAMILY OF B VITAMINS

The eight B vitamins are all water soluble. They are B_1 (thiamine), B_2 (riboflavin), B_3 (niacin), B_5 (pantothenate), B_6 (pyridoxine), B_7 (biotin), B_{12} (cobalamin), and folate. Although they have similar functions such as energy metabolism, neurotransmitter synthesis, fat and protein metabolism, nerve functions, brain health, and overall health, they each have unique functions as well. There is an interdependence among the B vitamins that renders the assessment of any one individual B vitamin flawed. If you were to evaluate the effectiveness of a hand by assessing the function of each digit, you could conclude that a hand is not very functional. The B vitamins are presented based upon their relationships and functions.

■ *4.4 The Busy Bs: B_1, B_2, B_3, B_5*
▶ VITAMIN B₁ (THIAMINE)

Thiamine was first isolated from rice bran as the factor that could prevent a severe neurological disorder called beriberi. The main thiamine coenzymes include thiamine diphosphate (TDP), also called thiamine pyrophosphate (TPP).

Functions
- Synthesis of nicotinamide adenine dinucleotide phosphate, a niacin-based reducing agent used in:
  - Anabolic reactions such as lipid and nucleic acid synthesis
  - Oxidation-reduction reactions that generate free radicals in immune cells for destruction of pathogens and protection against the toxicity of oxidation's reactive oxygen species
- Neurotransmitter synthesis: acetylcholine, GABA
- Energy transformation
- Glycolysis (the breakdown of glucose for energy)
- Carbohydrate metabolism
- Growth and development
- Nerve conduction
- Cardiac function

Risks for deficiency

- Inadequate intake
- Poor digestion (low gastric acid) and/or absorption
- Gastric bypass
- Anorexia
- Higher needs from illness, stress
- Refined foods
- Heated foods
- Medications: diuretics, Dilantin
- Consumption of raw fish

Deficiency disorders

- Beriberi (edema, tingling, burning sensations in hands and feet, confusion, trouble breathing, uncontrolled eye movements)
- Wernicke-Korsakoff syndrome from alcoholism or severe malnutrition (damaged brain and nerves, coordination problems, memory loss)
- Cardiac failure

Deficiency symptoms

- Sensory motor loss
- Loss of reflexes
- Foot/wrist drop
- Calf tenderness
- Confusion, memory problems
- Tongue glossitis (inflammation)
- Insomnia
- Headaches
- Myopathy (muscle weakness)
- Tachycardia (rapid heart rate)
- Enlarged heart
- Edema (swelling)
- Heart damage
- Pica (consumption of nonfood substances)
- Impaired vision
- Noise sensitivity
- Neuropathy

Thiamine and the Connection to ADHD and Autism

Optimal B vitamin status benefits overall health for everyone. The amount used for supplementation is not specific to ADHD and autism. It is always best, when able, to provide a B vitamin complex from 5 to 25 mg, to maintain balance in each individual B vitamin. The amount of thiamine present in a B complex or multiple vitamin may or may not be sufficient. When lab results indicate deficiency, therapeutic doses may be required and should be accomplished under the care of a practitioner.

The Busy Bs: Vitamin B$_1$

THIAMINE TOTAL DAILY GOAL DOSING

AGE	DOSE	FREQUENCY
2 to 5	5 to 10 mg	Daily with food before midday
6 to 10	10 to 20 mg	Daily with food before midday
11 +	25 mg	Daily with food before midday

▶ VITAMIN B₂ (RIBOFLAVIN)

Low intakes of riboflavin are common at all ages, but particularly in adolescents. Riboflavin has two coenzyme derivatives, flavin mononucleotide and flavin adenine dinucleotide, which are electron carriers and important in the production of the energy molecule ATP.

Functions
- Electron transport chain function (mitochondria)
- Fatty acid metabolism
- Purine metabolism
- Vitamin B_6 metabolism
- Niacin synthesis from tryptophan
- Choline metabolism
- Neurotransmitter metabolism: dopamine, tyramine, and histamine
- Glutathione/sulfation metabolism, via glutathione reductase
- Structure of secretory proteins
- DNA synthesis

Risks for deficiency
- Inadequate intake
- Poor digestion (low gastric acid) and/or absorption
- Higher needs from illness, stress
- Refined foods
- Heated foods
- Thyroid disorder
- Medications: diuretics

Deficiency disorders
- Severe seborrhea
- Acne rosacea
- Cornea vascularization (red eyes)
- Liver defects

Deficiency symptoms
- Fatigue
- Hair loss
- Dermatitis
- Growth delays
- Tongue glossitis (inflammation of papillae) and fissured tongue
- Cheilosis (i.e., cracks in the corner of the mouth)
- Burning, itching eyes

- Poor appetite
- Light sensitivity
- B_6 deficiency (B_2 is needed to convert B_6 to one of its active forms)
- Folate deficiency

Riboflavin and the Connection to ADHD and Autism

Riboflavin's role in ADHD and autism is related to its need in B_6 metabolism and function. Vitamin B_6 is important in many pathways and often found to be functionally deficient in autism and ADHD.

Riboflavin Supplements

- The forms used include riboflavin and riboflavin-5′-phosphate (R5P).

RIBOFLAVIN OR R5P TOTAL DAILY GOAL DOSING

AGE	DOSE	FREQUENCY
2 to 5	5 to 10 mg	Daily with food before midday
6 to 10	10 to 20 mg	Daily with food before midday
11 +	25 mg	Daily with food before midday

▶ VITAMIN B_3 (NIACIN, NIACINAMIDE)

Niacin is a generic term for nicotinic acid and niacinamide. Niacin was discovered through its deficiency disorder, pellagra, which was more prevalent in the Southern states where corn (which has an unavailable form of niacin) was a dietary staple. Niacin functions in the body as nucleotide forms: nicotinamide adenine dinucleotide (NAD+) and nicotinamide adenine dinucleotide phosphate (NADP+).

Vitamin activity is provided by both nicotinic acid and niacinamide. The difference between the two is that nicotinic acid, commonly called niacin, can cause a dilation of blood vessels resulting in a flushing around the upper chest and head. This effect has been used therapeutically to resolve headaches, but it can also be a bothersome side effect.

Tryptophan produces niacin and serotonin. The use of niacin spares tryptophan for more conversion to serotonin.

Functions
- Glycolysis (breaking down of glucose for energy)
- Energy metabolism
- Fatty acid metabolism
- Cholesterol and adenal steroid hormone synthesis
- Glutamate metabolism
- DNA repair
- Regeneration of glutathione and vitamin C

The Busy Bs: Vitamin B_2

The Busy Bs: Vitamin B_3

Risks for deficiency
- Inadequate intake
- Poor digestion (low gastric acid) and/or absorption
- Higher needs from illness, stress
- Refined foods
- Heated foods
- Alcohol
- Medications: diuretics, tetracycline, isoniazid, and antidepressants
- Reliance on corn as a staple

Deficiency disorders
- Pellagra: dermatitis, diarrhea, and dementia

Deficiency symptoms
- Fatigue
- "Red neck," as if sunburned
- Slow growth
- Tongue glossitis (inflamed papillae) and a sore tongue (Note: The sore tongue symptom is not found in the other B vitamin deficiencies.)
- Edema
- Weakness
- Diarrhea
- Skin conditions
- Mood disorders
- Hyperpigmentation of skin
- Elevated lipids
- Appetite loss
- Memory loss

Niacin and the Connection to ADHD and Autism

The role of serotonin support in ADHD and autism makes niacinamide an important supplement. Tryptophan converts to niacin as well as to serotonin and melatonin. By providing niacin, the tryptophan is spared to make more serotonin. Niacinamide itself is also important in energy metabolism and has a calming effect. Niacin has a long history of benefit in depression and more serious mental illnesses.

Niacin Supplements

We recommend only using niacinamide, the form of niacin that does not cause a flush. For higher doses or the use of niacin therapeutically for treating high cholesterol, consult with a physician.

NIACINAMIDE (NOT NIACIN) TOTAL DAILY GOAL DOSING

AGE	DOSE	FREQUENCY
2 to 5	25 mg	Daily with food
6 to 10	50 mg	Daily with food
11 +	100 mg	Daily with food

▶ VITAMIN B$_5$ (PANTOTHENATE, PANTOTHENIC ACID, AND CALCIUM PANTOTHENATE)

Pantothenic acid, known as vitamin B$_5$, is essential to all forms of life. The name comes from the Greek word *pantos*, meaning "everywhere." It is a component of coenzyme A (CoA), which is the active form of pantothenic acid. Pantethine is a derivative of pantothenic acid, which is also a component of CoA.

Pantothenic acid is one of the main nutrients termed "anti-stress." This likely stems from its numerous contributions to adrenal stability and function.

Functions
- Energy generated from protein, fat, and carbohydrates
- Synthesis of essential fatty acids, cholesterol, and steroid hormones
- Neurotransmitter synthesis (acetylcholine)
- Natural antihistamine
- Anti-stress nutrient
- Melatonin synthesis
- Cholesterol and triglyceride reduction (at doses of 900 mg/day)
- Adrenal support
- Synthesis of catecholamines
- Through its role in acetylation (the addition of acetate donated by CoA), there are numerous functions:
  - DNA replication
  - Cell division
  - Gene expression
  - Long chain fatty acid metabolism

Risks for deficiency
- Inadequate intake
- Poor digestion (low gastric acid) and/or absorption
- Higher needs from illness, stress
- Oral contraceptives
- Processed grains
- Diabetes
- Inflammation
- Alcohol
- Caffeine

Deficiency disorders
- Adrenal insufficiency
- Growth retardation
- Burning feet syndrome

Deficiency symptoms
- Fatigue
- Nausea
- Depression, anxiety
- Adrenal hypofunction
- Palpitations
- Poor healing
- Neuralgia
- Eczema
- Allergy (hives)
- Burning, tingling feet
- Toe walking
- Tooth grinding
- Insomnia
- Loss of hair pigment

Pantothenic Acid and the Connection to ADHD and Autism

Undermethylation is common in autism and a subset of those with ADHD, and is frequently associated with high histamine levels. Pantothenic acid has a strong antihistamine effect, rendering it ideal for those who are undermethylated *and* have symptoms of IgE allergies (runny nose, cough, itchy eyes, eczema, asthma, and dark circles under the eyes).

There is a subset of children with autism (less so in ADHD) that have weak adrenal function (adrenal hypofunction). Symptoms include pallor, weak muscles, dizziness upon standing quickly, poor endurance, and poor posture (slouching). Some may even experience fainting. Pantothenic acid supports adrenal function via acetyl-CoA conversion to HMG-CoA, the precursor to cholesterol, which is the parent of the adrenal steroid cortisol.

Pantothenic acid, vitamin C, amino acids, and biotin are an effective team in supporting healthy adrenal function.

Pantothenic Acid Supplements

For allergies, pantothenic acid is often taken along with vitamin C and quercetin, all three of which provide antihistamine and immune support without the side effects of the antihistamine medications. (See section 2.1 Allergies for dosing of vitamin C and quercetin.) Pantothenic acid is one of the safest supplements with no known toxicity at 20,000 mg or more daily.

PANTOTHENIC ACID TOTAL DAILY GOAL DOSING

AGE	DAILY DOSE	TOTAL DAILY DOSE
2 to 5	100 to 250 mg per day	250 mg
6 to 10	250 mg 2 or 3 times per day	750 mg
11 +	500 mg 2 times per day	1,000 mg

- Lower doses can be used for maintenance and reducing allergy potential.
- Antihistamine supplements should not be taken when being skin tested for allergies.

B VITAMINS: THIAMIN, RIBOFLAVIN, NIACIN, and PANTOTHENATE

VITAMIN	VITAMIN B₁ THIAMINE	VITAMIN B₂ RIBOFLAVIN	VITAMIN B₃ NIACIN NIACINAMIDE	VITAMIN B₅ PANTOTHENIC ACID
Diagnostic tests	Blood Tests ETK transketolase (High = deficient) Isoleucine (High = deficient) Urine Tests Isoleucine (High = deficient)	Blood Tests EGR (High = deficient) Urine Tests Ethyl malonate (High = deficient)	Urine Tests *N-Methylnicotinamide (High = deficient) Lactate (High = deficient) Pyruvate (High = deficient)	Serum Pantothenic Acid 1 to 10 years (Low = <200 ng/mL) (Normal = 200–1,241 ng/mL) (High = >1,241 ng/mL) Urine Tests Alpha-keto Acids (High = deficient) Urine pantothenate (Low = deficient)
Possible side effects	Irritability, increased activity	Irritability, increased activity	Flushing Stomach discomfort Diarrhea	Possible digestive symptoms at 2,000 mg or more
Toxicity	Nontoxic up to 500 mg/day	Nontoxic	Liver effects	Nontoxic Safe at doses in excess of 10,000 mg (10 grams)
Excess/toxicity side effects	Digestive upset	Digestive upset	Liver enzyme elevation Severe flushing Muscle pain, gout, jaundice Increased glucose, homocysteine	At 10 to 20 grams per day: diarrhea, nausea, heartburn
Food sources	Yeast, pork, sunflower seeds, legumes	Beef liver, steak, mushrooms, ricotta cheese, milk, oysters	Beef liver, fish, chicken, beef, mushrooms	Liver, kidney, meat, yolk, egg, yeast, broccoli, fish, legumes, whole grains, royal jelly, avocado
Interactions	*Enhancer:* alpha-lipoic acid *Antagonists:* diuretics, Dilantin	*Enhancers:* phosphorus, fiber *Antagonists:* oral contraceptives, tetracyclines, diuretics, UV light exposure	*Antagonists:* alcohol, diuretics, deficiencies of zinc, iron, B₆, and B₂ *Caution:* When taking high doses (over 500 mg), add B₁, B₂, and B₆.	*Enhancers:* vitamin C, other B vitamins *Antagonists:* alcohol, diuretics *Interferes with:* tetracyclines *Avoid in:* low histamine conditions

*Indicates most reliable tests

Vitamins B₁, B₂, B₃, B₅

■ 4.5 *The Worker Bs: Methylation Nutrients: Vitamin B₆, Methyl B₁₂, Folate, and DMG/ TMG*

Vitamins B_6 (pyridoxine), B_{12} (methylcobalamin), and folinic acid are water-soluble essential nutrients necessary for energy metabolism, and brain and nerve development and function. They are also critical participants in methylation, a process essential for regulating DNA synthesis, gene expression, enzymes, building neurotransmitters, synchronizing neuron firing, and creating cellular energy. For expanded information on methylation, refer to section 3.2 Mechanisms: Methylation. Dimethylglycine (DMG) and trimethylglycine (TMG) are methyl donors that also participate in methylation and support healthy neurotransmitter functions. These combined nutrient responsibilities profoundly affect cognition, focus, attention, language, energy metabolism, and development, all of which are important in ADHD and autism.

Methylation deficit is called undermethylation or hypomethylation. Excess methylation is called overmethylation or hypermethylation. Those who are undermethylated respond well to B vitamins, especially the methylation nutrients. Those who are over-methylated tend not to tolerate the methylation nutrients and can develop increased activity and irritability. See section 3.2 Mechanisms: Methylation.

Hypomethylation, according to William J. Walsh, Ph.D., Walsh Research Institute, occurs in:

- More than 95 percent of people with autism
- More than 99 percent of people with ADHD with an oppositional defiant presentation
- In 20 to 30 percent in other ADHD presentations

There is a significant interdependence among the B vitamins. For this reason, we usually recommend a B vitamin complex (separately or as part of a multiple vitamin–mineral), with the option to add additional individual B vitamins as indicated by symptoms and/or lab findings.

Testing for B_6, B_{12}, and folate should be accomplished by a skilled health care practitioner. Serum levels of these vitamins are not sensitive markers for deficiency and do not decline until extreme late stages of deficiency. There are specialized metabolite tests that are more specific for functions of all three.

▶ VITAMIN B₆ (PYRIDOXINE)

Vitamin B_6 is naturally present in many foods and added to others. There are six forms of B6: pyridoxine (PN), pyridoxal (PL), pyridoxamine (PM), pyridoxamine-5'-phosphate (PMP), pyridoxine-5'-phosphate (PNP), and the active form, pyridoxal-5'-phosphate (P5P). Substantial proportions of B_6 in grains, fruits, and vegetables are in a form that reduces their bioavailability. Vitamin B_6 (pyridoxine), as its active form P5P, affects more than 100 enzymes, especially those that depend upon magnesium.

Functions
- Cofactor for enzyme functions
- Amino acid, carbohydrate, and lipid metabolism
- Energy metabolism
- Hemoglobin and red blood cell formation
- Homocysteine regulation (along with magnesium, B_{12}, and folate as cofactors)
- Neurotransmitter biosynthesis
- Nerve function
- Steroid hormone metabolism
- Glucose control through gluconeogenesis (making of glucose) and glycogenolysis (breaking down of glycogen to make glucose)
- Immune modulation
- Niacin formation
- Nucleic acid synthesis

Risks for deficiency
- Inadequate intake
- Poor digestion and/or absorption
- Periods of higher energy demands: inflammation, trauma, growth, pregnancy, stress
- Depletion from medications: oral contraceptives, isoniazid, valproic acid
- Liver disease
- Excess protein intake (requires more B_6 as well as zinc)
- Smoke exposure (primary and secondhand)
- Environmental chemical exposures
- Caffeine
- Alcohol
- Impaired renal function
- Autoimmune disorder

Deficiency disorders
- Neuropathy
- Carpal tunnel syndrome
- Impaired gene expression

Deficiency symptoms
- Seborrheic dermatitis
- Tongue glossitis (inflammation) and/or fissures
- Cheilosis (angular cracks in the corner of the lips)
- Burning feet
- Irritability
- Mood disorders, depression, anxiety
- Confusion
- Poor cognition, attention, and focus
- Communication problems and language delays
- Fatigue

- Microcytic anemia (with possible coexisting iron and/or copper deficiency)
- Hyperactivity
- Inflammation
- Poor growth
- Neuralgia (nerve pain) or paresthesias (numbness and tingling)
- Muscle cramps
- Increased infections
- Premenstrual symptoms
- Hyperpigmentation (skin)
- Pregnancy nausea
- Homocysteinemia

Vitamin B_6 and the Connection to ADHD and Autism

In 1965, Bernard Rimland, Ph.D., investigated and promoted the use of vitamin B_6 as a therapy in autism, an idea then considered preposterous. The science caught up with him, and today vitamin B_6 is one of the most useful supplements in the treatment of ADHD and autism. It is effective in treating:

- Hyperactivity, excitability, self-stimulating behavior, anxiety, obsessive or repetitive behaviors

  B_6 is necessary for the enzyme glutamate decarboxylase to convert excitatory glutamate to calming GABA. An imbalance in glutamate and GABA is common in autism and may also be present in children with ADHD. GABA may be helpful in alleviating symptoms due to this imbalance.

- Cognition, attention, focus, communication, language, learning

  Vitamin B_6 (along with magnesium) impacts brain and neurological development and function leading to improved attention, cognition, focus, and communication.

- Mood, depression, anger

  Neurotransmitter metabolism is B_6 dependent, especially for serotonin, GABA, and dopamine pathways. These neurotransmitters are important in ADHD and autism.

Vitamin B_6 Supplements

A multiple vitamin–mineral or vitamin B complex may or may not provide sufficient doses of B_6 and/or its active coenzyme form pyridoxal-5′-phosphate (P5P.) If not sufficient, additional B_6 and/or P5P may be added.

VITAMIN B$_6$ OR P5P SUPPLEMENTS

SINGULAR B$_6$ OR P5P SUPPLEMENTS	INSTRUCTIONS
Vitamin B$_6$ 50 mg Hypoallergenic, made by *Kirkman Labs*	Start with ¼ capsule and increase as tolerated
P5P 30 mg, made by *Klaire Labs*	Start with ⅓ capsule and increase as tolerated
COMBINATION B$_6$ OR P5P WITH MAGNESIUM	INSTRUCTIONS
Klaire Labs P5P Plus (30 mg P5P + 100 mg Mg glycinate) made by *Klaire Labs*	Start with ⅓ capsule and increase as tolerated. This combination will meet the needs of the magnesium recommendations in this chapter.

VITAMIN B$_6$ AND P5P TOTAL DAILY GOAL DOSING

AGE	B$_6$ DOSE *DAILY WITH FOOD BEFORE MIDDAY*	P5P DOSE *DAILY WITH FOOD BEFORE MIDDAY*
2 to 5	10 to 15 mg	5 mg
6 to 10	20 to 30 mg	10 mg
11 +	50 mg	15 mg

- P5P is more potent than B$_6$ and usually given at lesser doses than B$_6$.
- B$_6$ and P5P are more effective if taken with magnesium.
- If sulfation is low, as is the case with phenol sensitivities/intolerances, avoid the P5P form of B$_6$ supplementation.
- Higher-than-recommended doses must be accomplished under the guidance of a health care practitioner.
- High doses given alone can cause peripheral neuropathy, which can be mitigated by other B vitamins and magnesium.
- Start at a lower dose and increase gradually.
- Discontinue if negative symptoms persist.

▶ VITAMIN B$_{12}$ (METHYLCOBALAMIN, METHYL B$_{12}$)

Vitamin B$_{12}$ is the most complex in structure of all the vitamins and contains the mineral cobalt, which is the cobalamin portion of all the forms of B$_{12}$. Although B$_{12}$ has such a significant influence on human health, only two enzymatic reactions have been identified in the body that are dependent upon B$_{12}$; one requires methylcobalamin and the other requires adenosylcobalamin.

Functions

- Methylation is one of the core processes in human metabolism. B$_{12}$ has a critical role in the methylation folate cycle. Methionine synthase (MS) conversion of homocysteine to methionine occurs in two steps:
  1. Cobalamin bound to MS picks up the methyl group from 5-methyltetrahydrofolate (5-MTHF) and transfers the methyl group from 5-MTHF forming THF and methylcobalamin bound to MS.

2. Methycobalmin bound MS releases the methyl group for transfer to homo-cysteine, producing methionine and MS-cobalamin.

Note: Without B_{12}, folate is trapped in the 5MTHF form.

- Energy metabolism:
  - L-methylmalonyl-CoA mutase (adenosyl B_{12} dependent) conversion of L-methylmalonyl-CoA to succinyl CoA
  - Succinyl CoA is part of the Krebs/citric acid cycle
    - Produces energy from fats and proteins
    - Is required in synthesis of hemoglobin (the oxygen-carrying pigment in the red blood cells)
    Note: When the mutase enzyme is impaired, methyl malonic acid (MMA) accumulates. This is the metabolite marker for B_{12} functional deficiency.
- Nucleic acid synthesis
- Neurological function—protection of myelin sheath covering of cranial, spinal, and peripheral nerves
- Neurotransmitter functions
- Hemoglobin and RBC formation

Risks for deficiency
- Inadequate intake or vegetarian/vegan diet
- Poor digestion (low gastric acid) and/or absorption
- Lack of intrinsic factor (needed for absorption)
- Pernicious anemia—an autoimmune condition that destroys gastric cells
- Atrophic gastritis—chronic inflammation and loss of acid and enzyme production
- Celiac disease
- Overgrowth of anaerobic bacteria from decreased stomach acid production
- Poor sulfation
- Gene variant defects in methylenetetrahydrofolate reductase—a frequent finding in autism
- Medications: antacids, diuretics, antiseizure medications, neomycin, and hormones
Note: Chronic use of antacids is a common cause of B_{12} deficiency of and other nutrients.

Deficiency disorders
- Neuropathy
- Neural tube defects due to impaired folate function secondary to B_{12} deficiency
- Failure to thrive
- Dementia

Deficiency symptoms
- Anemia: macrocytic, megaloblastic
- Neurological symptoms (neuropathy, numbness/tingling) from damage to myelin sheaths covering nerves (cranial, spinal, and peripheral)
- Fatigue
- Memory loss
- Abnormal gait, poor balance
- Growth retardation
- Developmental delays
- Mood disorders, depression
- RBC hemolysis
- Low monocyte levels
- Glossitis, loss of papillae (slick tongue)
- Inflammation from elevated homocysteine
- Tactile hypersensitivity (oversensitive to touch)
- Folic acid deficiency (from impaired methionine synthase)—folate gets trapped and methylation becomes impaired

Vitamin B$_{12}$ and the Connection to ADHD and Autism

Because undermethylation is found in more than 95 percent of those with autism, it is easy to understand why B$_{12}$ supplements are needed. B$_{12}$ improves cognition, communication, language, focus, attention, and energy.

B$_{12}$ deficiency is more prevalent in those with autism who have lymphonodular ileal hyperplasia (a problem in the small intestinal lining seen in some children with autism).

See Section 3.2 A: Methylation for more details on B$_{12}$ and methylation.

B$_{12}$ as Methylcobalamin Supplements

Methylcobalamin is preferred over cyanocobalamin, the most commonly used form. Cyanocobalamin must convert to methylcobalamin, a process that may not be efficient. A multiple vitamin–mineral or vitamin B complex may or may not provide sufficient doses of methylcobalamin. If not, additional methylcobalamin may be added.

Types of B$_{12}$ Supplements

- Oral (capsules, liquids, powders, and tablets)
- Sublingual (given under the tongue; helpful in absorption problems)— tablets or sprays
- Nasal spray or gel (helpful in absorption problems)
- Topical (helpful in absorption problems)
- Subcutaneous injections (best for therapeutic effects in some children— must be prescribed and monitored by a physician)

METHYL B$_{12}$ TOTAL DAILY GOAL DOSING

AGE	DOSE	FREQUENCY *TAKE WITH FOOD*	TOTAL DAILY DOSE FROM ALL SOURCES
2 to 5	50 to 100 mcg	Daily before noon	100 mcg
6 to 10	100 to 500 mcg	Daily before noon	500 mcg
11 +	500 to 1,000 mcg	Daily before noon	1,000 mcg

- To keep the dosing in the lower range, give a portion of the dose recommended on the label.

▶ FOLATE: FOLINIC ACID, 5-MTHF

Folate is water soluble and the generic term for all of the folate forms. Folic acid is synthesized and artificial. It is found in supplements and added to fortified foods. We prefer not to use folic acid as a supplement. It must convert to active tetrahydrofolate, and the conversion can be problematic. Folinic acid and 5-methyltetrahydrofolate (5-MTHF) are the physiologically active compounds and preferred for supplementation.

Functions
- Methylation (folate is the main factor in the folate cycle)
- Cell production and maintenance
- Production of DNA and RNA, the building blocks of cells
- Red blood cell and hemoglobin production

Risks for deficiency
- Inadequate intake
- Poor digestion (low gastric acid) and/or absorption
- B$_{12}$ deficiency (which causes problems in the folate cycle)
- Excessive tissue demand: illness, pregnancy, trauma, stress, alcoholism
- Defects in folate metabolism
- Methylenetetrahydrofolate reductase mutation
- Medications: antacids, diuretics, antiseizure medications, tetracycline, and methotrexate

Deficiency disorders
- Neural tube defects
- Neuropathy
- Mental retardation
- Homocysteinemia

Deficiency symptoms
- Anemia: macrocytic megaloblastic
- Neurological symptoms
- Cognitive decline
- Poor growth
- Fatigue
- Tongue: glossitis, loss of papillae

- Gingivitis (inflammation of the gums)
- Immune dysfunction
- Low monocytes
- Low white blood cell count
- Loss of villi in small intestine
- Diarrhea
- Cardiovascular diseases
- Cervical dysplasia
- Hyperpigmentation of skin
- In pregnancy: melasma and linea nigra (a dark line down the middle of the lower abdomen)
- Fetal/infant:
  - Failure to thrive
  - Developmental delays
  - Risk for autism spectrum disorders
  - Mental retardation

Folate and the Connection to ADHD and Autism

Because undermethylation is found in more than 95 percent of those with autism, the importance of folate is clear. In conjunction with B_{12}, there can be improvement in focus, attention, language, cognition, and behavior.

Folate Supplements

A multiple vitamin–mineral or vitamin B complex may or may not provide the right form of and/or sufficient doses of folate. If not, additional folate may be added.

Types of folate supplements
- Folinic acid is one of the preferred folate forms noted for its excellent bioavailability.
- Folic acid is least effective, can be problematic, and is best avoided.

SUPPLEMENT	INSTRUCTIONS
Folinic Acid 400 mcg Hypoallergenic, made by *Kirkman Labs*	Start with ¼ capsule and increase as tolerated
Combination: Folinic Acid with B_{12} Hypoallergenic 400 mcg folinic acid + 6 mcg methyl $B_{12,}$ made by *Kirkman Labs*	Start with ¼ capsule and increase as tolerated

FOLINIC ACID TOTAL GOAL DOSING

AGE	DOSE	FREQUENCY	TOTAL DAILY DOSE FROM ALL SOURCES
2 to 5	100 mcg	Daily	100 mcg
6 to 10	200 mcg	Daily	200 mcg
11 +	400 mcg	Daily	500 mcg

Methylation Cofactors: Dimethylglycine (DMG) and Trimethylglycine (TMG)

DMG and TMG both have methyl groups attached to the amino acid glycine and are both methyl donors, which are useful in undermethylation conditions. DMG has two methyl groups while TMG has three. These supplements have both been demonstrated to improve language, cognition, and eye contact, and to reduce echolalia, anxiety, and obsessive–compulsive behaviors. Not all individuals tolerated DMG and/or TMG.

The following information is helpful in achieving success with the addition of DMG or TMG:

DMG
- It is ideal to include folinic acid first.
- If folate function is insufficient, DMG may cause increased irritability, stimming, or hyperactivity.
- DMG can have a positive effect on speech, eye contact, and cognition

TMG
- When TMG donates a methyl group, it becomes DMG.
- TMG can produce positive results on speech and eye contact.
- If TMG results in side effects, adding taurine may improve tolerance.

DMG AND TMG TOTAL DAILY GOAL DOSING

SUPPLEMENT	AGE	DOSE	FREQUENCY	TOTAL DAILY DOSE FROM ALL SOURCES
DMG	2 to 5	125 mg	1 time per day	125 mg
	6 to 10	125 mg	2 times per day	250 mg
	11 +	250 mg	2 times per day	500 mg
TMG	2 to 5	175 mg	2 times per day	350 mg
	6 to 10	250 mg	2 times per day	500 mg
	11 +	500 mg	2 times per day	1,000 mg

- Some children respond better to TMG than DMG and vice versa.
- Higher doses must be accomplished under the guidance of a practitioner.

METHYLATION VITAMINS: PYRIDOXINE, METHYLCOBALAMIN, and FOLATE

VITAMIN	PYRIDOXINE VITAMIN B$_6$	METHYLCOBALAMIN VITAMIN B$_{12}$	FOLATE
Diagnostic tests	Urine Tests *Xanthurenate (High = deficient) *Kynurenate (High = deficient) Homocysteine (High = deficient) Blood Tests Plasma total homocysteine (High = deficient) Serum pyridoxine, P5P (Low = deficient) AST, ALT (Low = deficient)	Urine Tests *Methylmalonate (High = deficient) *Homocysteine (High = deficient) Blood Tests Plasma total homocysteine CBC with differential (MCV High = deficient) (MCH High = deficient) Serum B$_{12}$—not reliable	Urine Tests *FIGLU (High = deficient) *Homocysteine (High = deficient) Blood Tests Plasma total homocysteine (High = deficient) CBC with differential (MCV High = deficient) (MCH High = deficient) RBC Folate (Low = deficient) Serum folate—not reliable
Possible side effects	Irritability, increased activity	Irritability, increased activity	Irritability
Toxicity	Limited toxicity Use of 500 mg long term B$_2$ and R5P are protective	Broad range of safety in dosing	Not determined
Excess/toxicity side effects	Neuropathy (reversible)	Neuralgia (nerve pain) Anemia Folate deficiency	Neuralgia Anemia B$_{12}$ deficiency Masks B$_{12}$ deficiency
Food sources	Chickpeas, beef liver, fish, poultry, meat, fruit, vegetables	Animal source only: meats, especially beef liver; clams, fish, poultry, eggs, milk products	Green leafies, vegetables, beans, fruits, nuts
Interactions	B$_2$, magnesium, and zinc are required to convert B$_6$ to P5P *Enhancers:* magnesium, zinc phosphorus *Antagonists:* diuretics, antacids, caffeine, alcohol If sulfation is low, avoid P5P form of B$_6$	*Enhancers:* intrinsic factor, pepsin, gastric acid improve absorption Animal protein *Antagonists:* diuretics, antacids, celiac, antiseizure medications, alcohol	*Enhancers:* gastric acid, vitamin C, B$_5$, B$_{12}$, B$_6$, E Animal protein Folate requires B$_{12}$ for function *Antagonists:* alcohol, antiseizure medications, diuretic, antacids, tetracycline *Avoid in:* untreated B$_{12}$ pernicious anemia—it masks the symptoms

* Indicates most reliable tests

DMG and TMG

Biotin

■ 4.6 *The Helper B: Biotin*

Biotin is a water-soluble B vitamin. The major source is production by healthy GI flora. Bioavailability of biotin from foods is variable. Biotin maintains a healthy gut population (milieu) and is absorbed by the body for use in many important systemic functions. For a vitamin that is produced in such small amounts, it is a powerhouse in its effect on human health.

Functions

Biotin functions can overlap with those of zinc, vitamin A, vitamin D, and omega-3 essential fatty acids, especially regarding skin conditions and immunity.
- Energy metabolism
- Amino acid metabolism
- Synthesis of fatty acids for cell membranes
- Mitochondrial fatty acid oxidation
- Cholesterol metabolism
- Regulation of DNA replication and transcription
- Glucose control (gluconeogenesis)
- Immunity
- Neurological function
- Epithelial integrity: skin, mucosal tissues, and hair
- Cell growth
- Fetal and child growth and development

Causes of deficiency
- Genetic differences in enzymes involved in biotin metabolism
  - Biotinidase deficiency
  - Holocarboxylase synthetase deficiency (HCS)
  - Biotin transporter deficiency
- Insufficient healthy gut flora—results in poor production of biotin
- Poor intestinal absorption
- Chronic liver diseases, including cirrhosis
- Anticonvulsant medications such as Depakote or valproic acid
- Antibiotics, which depress biotin production, leading to yeast overgrowth
- Avidin, an antimicrobial protein, found in raw egg whites, which binds to biotin, preventing absorption; cooking the egg whites inactivates this effect
- Magnesium deficiency
- B_5 (pantothenic acid) deficiency

Deficiency disorders

Deficiencies of biotin, once considered rare, are now more prevalent, most likely due to poor gut flora and the widespread use of antibiotics.

Severe symptoms will occur from biotin-responsive metabolic or genetic conditions:
- Developmental delays
- Birth defects
- Failure to thrive
- Behavioral disorders
- Hypotonia
- Hearing loss
- Lack of coordination
- Learning disabilities
- Seizures
- SIDS
- Severe skin condition (acrodermatitis)

Deficiency signs and symptoms
- Hair loss (alopecia)
- Splitting fingernails
- Eczema
- Seborrheic dermatitis ("cradle cap" and scaly red rash around eyes, nose, mouth, and genital area)
- Unusual facial fat distribution (the characteristic facial rash and unusual facial fat distribution is termed the "biotin-deficient facies.")
- Yeast overgrowth and bowel dysbiosis
- Conjunctivitis
- Neurological symptoms/paresthesias
- Increased bacterial and fungal infections
- Immune deficiencies
- Muscle weakness
- Mood disorders
- Unusual urine odor

Note: The skin conditions associated with biotin deficiency are commonly misdiagnosed as eczema or dermatitis and treated with topical creams. The symptoms of biotin deficiency can overlap with deficiency symptoms of zinc, vitamin A, vitamin D, and omega-3 fatty acids. The most successful (and safe) treatments are those that address the underlying issues and incorporate the full complement of nutrients.

Biotin and the Connection to ADHD and Autism
Imbalances in gut flora including yeast overgrowth are common among children who have had repeat courses of antibiotics for recurrent infections. Antibiotics deplete biotin-synthesizing good flora leading to intestinal fungal overgrowth and systemic biotin deficiency, affecting immunity, skin health, development, and metabolism. Biotin helps keep yeast in a less invasive form, which makes it easier to eradicate.

BIOTIN TOTAL DAILY GOAL DOSING

AGE	DOSE	FREQUENCY
2 to 5	500 mcg to 5 mg	Daily
6 to 10	5 mg	Daily
11 +	5 to 10 mg	Daily

Higher doses should be accomplished only under the guidance of a skilled medical practitioner.

Biotin

BIOTIN

Tests	β-hydroxyisovalerate (urine) (High = deficiency) Vaccenic fatty acid (serum) (High = deficiency) Urinary biotin excretion (Reduced = deficiency) Plasma biotin—not reliable
Side effects	Possible constipation (if not taking magnesium)
Toxicity side effects	No toxicity reported up to 200 mg (highest dose studied)
Sources	Most abundant source is from colonic production by beneficial flora Foods: brewer's yeast, liver, egg yolk, Swiss chard, nuts, avocado, cauliflower, salmon, and sardines
Interactions	Biotin is synergistic with most B vitamins, especially B$_5$. At doses higher than 10 mg of biotin, magnesium should be supplemented

▪ 4.7 Vitamin C

Vitamin C (ascorbic acid) is an essential water-soluble vitamin with diverse functions and multiple benefits. Humans lack the enzyme L-gulonolactone oxidase, which is needed to produce ascorbic acid, rendering the vitamin an essential nutrient. Humans are therefore unable to increase production in times of stress or illness.

Initial recommended levels were designed to prevent scurvy, which causes severe bleeding gingivae (gums). The current limited RDAs only apply to most "healthy" people. More optimal levels support the immune system, protect the body from oxidative stress, reduce allergies, and support healthy bowel movements.

Functions
- Antioxidant
- Antihistamine
- Oxidation and reduction functions
- Immune support
- Vascular integrity
- Leukocyte (white blood cell) function
- Regeneration of vitamin E
- Healing collagen (important for wound healing)
- Synthesis of neurotransmitters (dopamine, serotonin)
- Synthesis of carnitine
- Improved absorption of nonheme iron

Risks for deficiency
- Inadequate intake
- Poor digestion and/or absorption
- Illness

- Trauma
- Inflammation
- Oxidative stress (see section 3.2 Mechanisms: Oxidation)
- Stress
- Caffeine
- Tobacco (smokers and secondhand smoke)
- Alcohol
- Sodas (diet and regular)
- Cortisone
- Diuretics
- Toxins

Deficiency disorders and associated conditions
- Scurvy
- Growth retardation

Deficiency signs and symptoms
- Capillary fragility, causing easy bruising or bleeding
- Immune dysfunction
- Poor bone healing
- Joint pain
- Dental problems: gingivitis, periodontitis
- Cataracts
- Depression, anxiety
- Anemia
- Folate deficiency

Vitamin C Supplements

We recommend using a supplement that only contains vitamin C. Some vitamin C products also contain other immune-supporting nutrients. It is best to use a pure vitamin C supplement as ascorbic acid to avoid potential overdosing of other nutrients that may be included. Note that some vitamin C supplements contain corn, which should be avoided if your child is allergic or sensitive to corn.

Vitamin C is contraindicated in the following conditions. Please consult with your child's physician.
- Kidney disease of any kind
- Oxalate kidney stone formation (increases with vitamin C use)
- Hemochromatosis (iron storage disease)
- G6PD deficiency (inherited blood disorder)

Dosing Information
- Vitamin C has an extremely wide dosing range and is found to be safe at doses as high as 10,000 mg.
- Vitamin C can be taken regularly at maintenance doses, with increases for allergic reactions, immune challenges, and illness.

Vitamin C

- The body self-regulates via "bowel tolerance" (the dose that does not cause diarrhea), the point at which absorption declines. This self-limiting makes toxicity very unlikely.

Vitamin C and the Connection to ADHD and Autism

Vitamin C can help treat constipation and allergies, both of which are not uncommon in children with ADHD and autism. For children with frequent infections or weak immune systems, vitamin C may be helpful. Children with autism may also have oxidative stress; vitamin C is an antioxidant. Recent research suggests a subset of individuals with autism may have difficulty synthesizing carnitine; vitamin C has a role in carnitine synthesis.

Immune issues, oxidative stress, and inflammation, which are common in people with autism, can increase the body's need for vitamin C beyond the RDA. The doses used are not intended to correct deficiency; they are used as therapy for the conditions.

Vitamin C Supplements in ADHD and Autism
Vitamin C Supplements
- Vitamin C 250 mg Hypoallergenic capsules, made by Kirkman Labs
- Pure ascorbic acid

VITAMIN C TOTAL DAILY GOAL DOSING

AGE	DOSE	FREQUENCY
2 to 5	100 to 250 mg	1 or 2 times per day
6 to 10	500 mg	1 or 2 times per day
11 +	500 to 1,000 mg	1 or 2 times per day

- Start at half of the lowest recommended dose and increase as tolerated.
- Watch for possible side effects and decrease the dose accordingly.
- If symptoms improve at lower than the goal dose, you may not need to continue to increase the dose.
- Do not exceed these recommended doses without the guidance of a health care practitioner.

VITAMIN C TOTAL DAILY GOAL DOSING FOR CONSTIPATION

AGE	DOSE	FREQUENCY
2 to 5	250 to 500 mg	1 or 2 times per day
6 to 10	500 mg	1 or 2 times per day
11 +	1,000 mg	1 or 2 times per day

VITAMIN C TOTAL DAILY GOAL DOSING FOR ALLERGIES

AGE	MAINTENANCE DOSE	INCREASE FOR ALLERGIES
2 to 5	100 mg per day	100 mg 2 or 3 times per day
6 to 10	250 mg per day	250 mg 2 or 3 times per day
11 +	500 mg per day	500 mg 2 times per day

VITAMIN C ASCORBIC ACID

Tests	Plasma vitamin C Urine ascorbic acid (available through specialty labs)
Possible side effects	Diarrhea, gas, abdominal cramps, nausea
Toxicity	Low toxicity; not believed to cause serious adverse effects at intakes as high as 10,000 mg
Toxic/excess side effects	Diarrhea Kidney stones Copper deficiency
Sources	Vegetables and fruits
Interactions	*Enhancers:* bioflavonoids, L-carnitine *Antagonists:* oxidants, diuretics, caffeine, steroids, illness, stress, inflammation, toxins Vitamin C increases iron absorption, which is beneficial if iron is low, but it should be avoided if iron is excessive.

MINERALS
■ 4.8 *Magnesium and Calcium*

Magnesium is a mineral that plays a role in more than 350 important metabolic reactions in the body. These include energy production, synthesis of essential molecules, hormone metabolism, neurotransmitter function, and cell signaling. Most of the functions of ATP (adenosine triphosphate—the body's energy molecule) require magnesium. Magnesium deficiency is common in children with ADHD and with autism. Magnesium can be helpful in the treatment of hyperactivity, anxiety, irritability, mood regulation, inattention, muscle cramps, constipation, hormonal imbalances, and sleep disruption, to name but a few of its myriad benefits.

Approximately 99 percent of total body magnesium is intracellular (inside cells); only 1 percent is extracellular. Blood testing inside the red blood cell (RBC magnesium) is therefore more reliable than serum magnesium.

Functions
- Cofactor for more than 350 enzyme functions
- Metabolism of carbohydrates and fats
- Involved in synthesis of protein and nucleic acid (DNA and RNA)
- Methylation metabolism
- Sulfur amino acid metabolism
- Glutathione metabolism

Magnesium and Calcium

- Transport of calcium and potassium across cell membranes
- Affects nerve impulse conduction, normal heart rhythm, and muscle contraction
- Important in potassium status
- Part of the structure of bone, cell membranes, and chromosomes
- Hormone metabolism
- Formation of active cofactor vitamins B_1, B_2, B_3, B_6, and pantothenate (B_5)
- Neuromuscular function
- Neurotransmitter function
- ATP production
- Formation of cAMP, a cell-signaling molecule

Causes of deficiency
- Inadequate intake
- Poor digestion and/or absorption
- Kidney disorders (magnesium wasting)
- Antacids
- Diuretics
- Caffeine
- Alcohol
- Phytates in fiber
- Laxative overuse/abuse
- Excess calcium

Deficiency disorders/diseases
- Seizures
- Preeclampsia and toxemia in pregnancy
- Sudden infant death syndrome (SIDS)
- Osteoporosis
- Arrhythmias (abnormal heart rhythms) or cardiac vasospasm

Deficiency signs and symptoms
- Muscle cramps
- Insomnia, sleep disruption, restless sleep
- Hyperactivity
- Anxiety
- Constipation
- Excessive sighing or yawning
- Tics
- Tremor
- Neuromuscular excitability, easy startle, brisk reflexes
- Salt craving
- Mood dysregulation including depression and irritability
- Memory loss
- High blood pressure
- Low potassium

Magnesium and the Connection to ADHD and Autism

Children with ADHD and autism often have multiple symptoms that can be seen with magnesium deficiency. You will note how often magnesium is mentioned under the symptom discussions in chapter 2. Green leafy vegetables, a main dietary source of magnesium, are not usually large components of a typically developing child's diet; children with autism who often have very picky appetites are at even greater risk for inadequate intake.

Magnesium Supplements

The type of magnesium used often depends on whether you are also trying to treat constipation. Magnesium tends to have laxative effects. Different forms of magnesium have more or less of this effect. Magnesium citrate has more laxative effect while magnesium glycinate, chelates, and gluconates have less laxative effect. Magnesium citrate has a stronger taste and some children may refuse it.

Magnesium supplements come in different forms (citrate, gluconate, glycinate, chelate, aspartate, and more). The elemental amount of magnesium in each compound varies according to the compound. For example, in 500 mg of magnesium glycinate, the elemental amount is 50 mg. The dose of magnesium refers to the elemental amount of magnesium in the compound.

MAGNESIUM SUPPLEMENTS

WELL TOLERATED, GENTLE STOOL EFFECT GOOD BIOAVAILABILITY	LAXATIVE STOOL EFFECT GOOD BIOAVAILABILITY	MIXED STOOL EFFECT POOR BIOAVAILABILITY
Magnesium chelate (sweet, sandy)	Magnesium citrate (salty, sandy)	Magnesium sulfate (laxative) (strong taste)
Magnesium aspartate (slightly bitter, salty)	Magnesium chloride (salty)	Magnesium oxide (firms stools) (chalky, neutral)
Magnesium glycinate (neutral)		
Magnesium gluconate (tangy)		

MAGNESIUM TOTAL DAILY GOAL DOSING

AGE	DOSE	FREQUENCY	TOTAL DAILY DOSE FROM ALL SOURCES
2 to 5	100 mg	1 or 2 times per day	200 mg
6 to 10	100 mg	2 or 3 times per day	300 mg
11 +	100 to 150 mg	2 or 3 times per day	450 mg

- Start at one-quarter to one-half of the recommended dose and increase the dose gradually every one to two days.
- Magnesium can cause loose stools or diarrhea.
- Watch for possible side effects and decrease the dose accordingly.

Magnesium and Calcium

- If symptoms improve at a lower dose, you may not need to continue to increase the dose.
- For higher-than-recommended doses, consult with a health care practitioner.

Calcium

Make sure calcium intake, either through diet or supplement, is adequate. Magnesium and calcium are inversely related, meaning that excess magnesium intake can lower calcium, and excess calcium intake can lower magnesium. It is important to have balance. If your child is on a milk/casein-free diet or not getting sufficient calcium from diet, a calcium supplement is indicated.

Calcium taken without adequate magnesium can result in poor calcium utilization, muscle cramping, constipation, joint pain, and an increase in ectopic calcifications including kidney stones. Calcium enhances contractions, while magnesium enhances muscle relaxation. The ratio of calcium to magnesium should be at least 2:1, and for some with high magnesium needs, the ratio is 1:1.

Enhancers to calcium include vitamin D_3, magnesium, vitamin B_6, boron, essential fatty acids, vitamin K, taurine, and protein.

Antagonists include excess protein, diuretics, caffeine, sodas, antacids, excessive fiber, toxic metals, and tetracyclines.

CALCIUM TOTAL DAILY GOAL DOSING

AGE	DOSE	FREQUENCY	TOTAL DAILY DOSE FROM ALL SOURCES
2 to 5	250 mg	2 times per day	500 mg
6 to 10	250 mg	3 times per day	750 mg
11 +	500 to 600 mg	2 times per day	1,000 to 1,200 mg

MAGNESIUM

Tests	Red blood cell magnesium, not serum magnesium Hair testing
Possible side effects	Gas, diarrhea
Toxicity side effects	Toxicity for oral intake is rare in individuals with normal kidney function. Magnesium is self-limiting in that the diarrhea results in a loss of magnesium. Diarrhea, low blood pressure, lethargy, confusion, low calcium, abnormal cardiac rhythm, muscle weakness, difficulty breathing
Sources	Green leafy vegetables, chlorophyll, unrefined grains "Hard" mineral water
Interactions	*Enhancers:* vegetable-based diet, B_6, vitamin D_3 *Synergisms:* magnesium-containing antacids and laxatives *Antagonists:* diuretics, antacids, laxatives, caffeine, alcohol, antibiotics, poor absorption, excess calcium, phosphorus *Avoid in:* hypocalcemia (low blood calcium), end stage renal disease (ESRD)

■ *4.9 Zinc*

Zinc is the second most common mineral in the body and found in every cell. Zinc's importance is evident by the long listing of its myriad functions and the symptoms that can result from its deficiency. Zinc deficiency is extremely common in individuals with autism and can be seen in children with ADHD.

Functions
There are more than 300 zinc-dependent enzyme functions:
- Energy metabolism
- Gene expression
- Immunity and thymus health
- Wound healing
- Cell growth
- Development and growth
- White blood cell development
- Protein and collagen development
- Alkaline phosphatase function
- SOD (antioxidant) function
- Insulin structure
- Digestive enzyme structure
- Brain pruning and function
- Sensory development
- Appetite and taste perception
- Vision development and function
- Language
- Metallothionein function (zinc and copper regulation, toxic metal detoxification, and protection against reactive oxygen species)
- Toxic metal antagonism
- Vitamin A transport through retinal binding protein
- Vitamin D regulation
- Amino acid metabolism
- Epithelial (skin, mucosal) health

Risks for deficiency
- Inadequate intake
- Poor digestion and/or absorption
- Medications/drugs: antacids, diuretics, steroids, antibiotics, hormone therapy, alcohol, and metal chelating agents
- Toxics: copper, lead, cadmium, and mercury
- Nutrients: excessive intake of calcium, iron, and copper
- Diarrhea
- Celiac disease
- Crohn's disease
- Intestinal parasites
- Sickle cell disease
- Bariatric surgery

Zinc

- Alcoholism
- Autism-related enterocolitis
- Poor insulin structure and function, diabetes
- Chronic kidney disease
- Chronic liver disease
- Stress
- Diet:
  - Glycemic (sugar-raising) diet. Zinc is part of the insulin molecule and is used up more rapidly when blood sugar is continually raised.
  - Vegan and vegetarian foods have a lower bioavailability of zinc due to the high phytate content of beans and grains, which bind zinc, iron, calcium, and magnesium.

Deficiency disorders
- Acrodermatitis enteropathica (metabolic disorder causing impaired uptake of zinc): severe dermatitis around the mouth, anus, and on the skin; alopecia (hair loss); diarrhea

Deficiency signs and symptoms
- Developmental delays
- Poor immunity and wound healing
- Chronic infections
- Poor cognition
- Inattention
- Eczema, dermatitis, acne
- Infertility
- Poor muscle tone
- White lines on nails
- Night blindness
- Hair loss
- Hypothyroidism
- Toxic metal accumulation
- Sensory symptoms: vision, auditory, smell, touch, taste
- Loss of taste, smell, appetite
- Food aversions (especially to vegetables)
- Pica (eating nonfood substances)
- Low salivary gustin
- Poor eye contact and vision dysfunction
- Poor oral motor tone
- Speech and communication delays
- Poor amino acid utilization
- Vitamin A deficiency (secondary to zinc deficiency)

RECOMMENDED ZINC ORAL SUPPLEMENTS (LIQUIDS, CAPSULES, AND POWDERS)

NUTRIENT FORM	TASTE	SIDE EFFECTS INSTRUCTIONS
Zinc gluconate	Neutral taste	Well tolerated
Zinc citrate	Tangy and sour	Avoid if citrate levels are high
Zinc picolinate	Bitter	Tolerance varies
Zinc chelates	Neutral to sour	
Zinc acetate	Sour, salty	
Zinc sulfate liquid	Strong taste (sulfur) Needs to be disguised	Stomach discomfort Disguise well Take with food
Zinc chloride liquid	Neutral taste	Well tolerated

Not recommended:
- Zinc oxide: poor bioavailability and can combine with other compounds to form insoluble complexes
- Zinc carbonate: poorly absorbed with poor bioavailability

Topical/Transdermal Lotions
Zinc lotions are available commercially and through compounding pharmacies. We prefer zinc sulfate because most children with autism need sulfate to improve toxin removal. Kirkman Labs (www.kirkmanlabs.com) is one resource for a commercially available zinc lotion that contains 22 mg of zinc per scoop (⅛ teaspoon).

It is best to apply the lotion to parts of the body that have more muscle than fat. Muscle has a rich blood supply that enhances the absorption. Apply the lotion to shoulders, back, or calves and massage in thoroughly.

When using more than one transdermal supplement lotion, it is best not to mix them together. They can be applied at the same time on different parts of the body.

Zinc and Copper
Zinc and copper are mutually antagonistic: Excesses of one can lower the other. Copper is an important nutrient for many reactions in the body, however, it tends to be higher in those with autism and less so in ADHD. Testing through a health care practitioner is critical prior to supplementing with copper. At higher levels of zinc, copper levels should also be monitored to avoid deficiency.

Some multivitamins also contain zinc; the amount varies greatly. Be careful not to exceed the total daily dose between the combination of a multivitamin and separate zinc supplement.

Zinc and the Connection to ADHD and Autism
Zinc deficiency is extremely common in children with autism and can also be seen in children with ADHD. A very common consequence in both disorders is picky eating, which can be due to impaired taste perception caused by zinc

deficiency. Zinc is necessary for retinol-binding protein, the carrier for vitamin A. In children with autism, vitamin A deficiency caused by zinc deficiency can contribute to poor eye contact. Zinc has such widespread effects on biochemistry and subsequent symptoms that treating deficiency can result in improvements in a variety of areas.

ZINC TOTAL DAILY GOAL DOSING

AGE	DOSE	FREQUENCY	TOTAL DAILY DOSE FROM ALL SOURCES
2 to 5	5 to 10 mg	1 or 2 times per day	10 to 20 mg
6 to 10	10 mg	2 times per day	20 mg
11 +	10 to 15 mg	1 or 2 times per day	20 to 30 mg

- Without testing, these ranges should not be exceeded without the advice of a health care practitioner.
- For optimal absorption, an empty stomach is best, but this may not be feasible if nausea occurs. Large doses can cause gastric discomfort and nausea and inhibit the digestive enzyme DPP-IV, which digests opioids from gluten and casein.
- Avoid or limit giving zinc at the same time as interfering nutrients: calcium, iron, folate, and phosphorylated nutrients (R5P, P5P, phosphatidylcholine); this may not always be feasible.
- Zinc excess can lower copper levels. Copper levels need to be maintained.
- Utilize the Zinc Tally Taste Test for evaluating progress with zinc supplementation. See page 213.
- Higher doses may be required due to malabsorption, antacid use, toxic metals, or lab findings. This should be accomplished with a skilled health care practitioner.

ZINC

Tests	Red blood cell zinc, not serum zinc RBC zinc is much more sensitive Zinc Tally Taste Test Hair
Possible side effects	Nausea (most common side effect) Absorption is best on an empty stomach, but may cause upset
Toxicity	150 to 450 mg long term
Toxic/excess side effects	Headaches, nausea, vomiting, cramps, abdominal pain Metallic taste Low WBC Anemia due to copper deficiency High cholesterol and low LDL
Sources	Seafood, oysters, meat, liver, milk
Interactions	*Enhancers:* B vitamins, pancreatic enzymes, animal protein, picolinate, citrate *Antagonists:* Antacids, diuretics, malabsorption, excess copper, toxic metals Can interfere with DPP-IV enzyme, which digests opiate-like peptides Avoid use in Menkes disease (genetic copper deficiency disorder).

Screening Test for Zinc

The taste test for zinc, the Zinc Tally Taste Test by Metagenics, is a weak solution of zinc sulfate. The better the zinc status, the stronger the taste.

Zinc Tally Taste Test Directions
- Give the liquid at least a half an hour after food or any drink so that taste buds are clear.
- For children, give 1 teaspoon.
- For adults, give 2 teaspoons.
- Adults or older children can swish the liquid around in the mouth for ten seconds and then spit it out.
- Younger children can swallow the liquid, as the goal is to coat the taste buds.
- Observe the child's immediate reaction in the first ten seconds.

ZINC TALLY TASTE TEST INTERPRETATION

TASTE WITHIN 10 SECONDS	INTERPRETATION
No taste or tastes like water	Deficient
Slight taste of something mild	Moderate
Strong offensive taste (metallic sulfur)	Good

Regardless of Zinc Tally Taste Test results, we would recommend not exceeding dosing amounts shown in the previous chart without blood testing.

■ *4.10 Selenium*

Selenium is a trace element that is required by the body in small amounts but can be toxic in large amounts. Selenium is used in the synthesis of selenoproteins, which are important antioxidant enzymes. Selenium requires methylation for metabolism. Selenium is unique in that it can substitute for sulfur in cysteine creating selenocysteine, important in many processes including metabolism, antioxidant functions (glutathione peroxidase), detoxification, and methionine metal metabolism (e.g., zinc, copper, and cadmium).

Functions
- Antioxidant: prevents cellular damage from free radicals
- Sulfation
- Regulates thyroid function
- Improves immune function
- Cardiovascular health
- Liver function
- Gastrointestinal health
- Musculoskeletal function

Selenium

Selenium and the Connection to ADHD and Autism

Individuals with autism may have oxidative stress, a condition in which toxic by-products of metabolism called free radicals may be in excess, with the potential to damage cell walls and ultimately DNA. Selenium is a good antioxidant. Selenium can be depleted by toxic metals, which are a problem in a subset of children with autism.

Selenium Supplements

Because of selenium's unique ability to substitute for sulfur in cysteine, it can be helpful in low sulfation conditions, which tend to be common in autism and to a lesser degree in ADHD. The inclusion of selenium as a supplement for ADHD and autism is important for two reasons:
- Sulfation and antioxidant benefit
- Prevention of selenium deficiency as a result of high zinc supplementation

Selenium dosing is best done under the guidance of a health care practitioner.

AMINO ACIDS
■ 4.11 *GABA and Theanine*

Children with autism, and possibly children with ADHD, may have imbalances in the brain between excitotoxic and calming transmitters. Excitotoxins make the brain cells fire excessively, which can be damaging to the cells. The brain tries to achieve a balance between excitation and inhibition (calming) in the brain. When there is increased excitation, excitatory glutamate converts to calming gamma-aminobutyric acid (GABA) to keep this balance. (See Section 3.1 D: The Neurologic System.) When this balance is disrupted, behavioral symptoms can develop and death or damage to brain cells may occur. The enzyme responsible for converting glutamate to GABA uses vitamin B_6 as a cofactor for its activity, so B_6 deficiency, common in autism, can also be a contributing factor to this imbalance.

Excess glutamate is found in:
- Additives such as MSG
- Foods containing high glutamate (processed foods, cow's milk products, whey, casein, wheat gluten, meats, fish, corn protein, soy protein, gelatin, broths, bouillon, and extracts)
- Medications and foods containing aspartame (diet sodas, junk food, diet foods, chewable tablets and gummies)

Potentially helpful supplements for improving the glutamate/GABA imbalance and improving symptoms include GABA and L-theanine.

GABA

GABA is an amino acid that functions as an inhibitory (calming) transmitter in the brain. There is debate about whether GABA is too large a molecule to be able to cross the blood–brain barrier. However, brain permeability can be affected by a number of factors, as outlined in Section 3.1 D: The Neurologic System. In the setting of increased permeability of the blood–brain barrier, it may be possible for GABA to cross into the brain. The effects are attributed to GABA neurotransmitter function. Vitamin B_6 is critical to GABA function, and B_6 deficiency is common in autism and also in ADHD. It is our clinical experience that GABA is helpful in up to 50 percent of patients.

Potential benefits from GABA
- Increased language
- Increased attention
- Decreased hyperactivity
- Decreased anxiety, OCD, repetitive or perseverative behaviors

Possible side effects include irritability or worsened behavior and sleepiness. Interactions include:
- Caffeine (increases glutamate activity and inhibits GABA release)
- Alcohol (decreases glutamate activity and increases GABA release)
- Taurine (increases GABA receptors)

GABA Supplements
- GABA is absorbed best on an empty stomach, which may not be feasible. It may be taken with food.
- GABA's beneficial effects may affect dosing of medications used for ADHD, anxiety, and seizures. Do not add GABA without discussing it with your child's physician.
- GABA should not be used if a child is already taking a medication that increases or potentially affects GABA such as benzodiazepines, barbiturates, narcotics, and gabapentin.
- GABA, especially at high doses, should only be used under the guidance of a health care practitioner.

GABA TOTAL DAILY GOAL DOSING

AGE	DOSE	FREQUENCY	TOTAL DAILY DOSE FROM ALL SOURCES
2 to 5	25 to 50 mg	2 times per day (breakfast and dinner)	50 to 100 mg
6 to 10	50 to 100 mg	2 times per day (breakfast and dinner)	100 to 200 mg
11 +	250 mg	1 or 2 times per day (breakfast and dinner)	250 to 500 mg

L-Theanine
L-theanine is an amino acid small enough to cross the blood–brain barrier. Its primary effect is to increase the level of GABA in the brain. It can also increase dopamine, which is important in ADHD. Potential side effects include:
- Irritability or worsened behavior

GABA and Theanine

- Sleepiness
- Decreased blood pressure. Use caution if taking with blood pressure medication.

L-theanine supplements
- The same caveats exist for L-theanine as were described for GABA.
- We recommend that you not use L-theanine without the guidance of a health care practitioner.

L-THEANINE TOTAL DAILY GOAL DOSING

AGE	DOSE	FREQUENCY	TOTAL DAILY DOSE FROM ALL SOURCES
2 to 5	50 mg	1 or 2 times per day (breakfast and dinner)	50 to 100 mg
6 to 10	100 mg	1 or 2 times per day (breakfast and dinner)	100 to 200 mg
11 +	200 mg	1 or 2 times per day (breakfast and dinner)	200 to 400 mg

■ *4.12 Taurine*

Taurine is a sulfur-containing "conditionally essential" amino acid, meaning it can be manufactured by the body. It is made in the liver and concentrated in muscle and the central nervous system. Taurine can be made from the amino acid cysteine when vitamin B_6 is adequate.

Functions
- Improves magnesium cellular uptake and utilization
- Protects against glutamate toxicity by regulating the balance between glutamate and GABA in the brain
- Antioxidant
- Conjugates (combines) with bile acids, which eliminate fat-soluble wastes
- May enhance bile flow and increase cholesterol clearance by liver
- Participant in a liver detoxification process known as phase II glucuronidation and sulfation (refer to section 3.2 Mechanisms: Sulfation)
- Facilitates uptake of essential fats and fatty acids from the small intestine
- Helps stabilize membranes (e.g., in the heart, brain, and muscles)
- Stabilizes platelets against aggregation
- Eye health: important in the retina via antioxidant properties and maintaining the structure and function of photoreceptor cells
- May act as an antianxiety agent in the brain by activating the glycine receptor

Risks for deficiency
- Inadequate intake
- Poor absorption
- Vegetarian or vegan diet

- Vitamin B_6 deficiency (B_6 is necessary for taurine's synthesis from cysteine)
- Zinc deficiency, resulting in increased urine taurine levels

Deficiency signs and symptoms
- Constipation
- Yellow or gritty/sandy stools
- Poor sleep
- Seizures
- Low levels of fat-soluble vitamins (A, D, E, K)
- Night blindness

Taurine and the Connection to ADHD and Autism

Taurine has many possible benefits, particularly for children with autism. It can be helpful in easing constipation because of its role in bile produced in the liver as conjugated bile salts, which are stored in the gallbladder. Prior to secretion, bile acids are combined (conjugated) with taurine or glycine and are released in the form of bile salts, the most common of which contains taurine (taurocholic acid). In response to fat intake, bile is released from the gallbladder into the small intestine to assist in fat digestion and absorption. Bile promotes intestinal motility; insufficient or ineffective bile can contribute to constipation. Bile also gives stools their normal brown color. When there is not enough bile, stools may be yellow or light colored. They may also appear sandy or gritty due to bile salts that have not bound to taurine.

Taurine also improves magnesium function. This can result in a calming effect, both due to taurine's direct influence on GABA and by enhancing magnesium function. Taurine may be helpful for lowering anxiety and treating motor tics. Taurine also has antiseizure benefits.

An increase in excitotoxins (glutamate) and reduction of calming transmitters (GABA) in the brain has been identified in many children with autism. (See Section 3.1 D: The Neurologic System for details.) Taurine helps counter high glutamate activity by activating GABA receptors.

Excessive toxin exposure is a concern in both children with autism and ADHD, given the general toxin exposure from our environment (see Section 3.2 B: Sulfation for details). Taurine has a major role in detoxification. Taurine conjugates with cholesterol to form bile acids, through which most fat-soluble toxins and wastes are eliminated.

Chronic inflammation in the brain or intestine can also be present, particularly in children with autism. In the presence of persistent inflammation and oxidative stress, cysteine, from which taurine is made, can be shunted away from taurine formation and used for making glutathione. Glutathione supports detoxification and is an important antioxidant.

If glutamate increases, as in the imbalanced state seen in the brain of many children with autism, taurine may increase as a compensatory mechanism to help protect the brain.

Taurine

Taurine Dosing

We would recommend not using taurine without the guidance of a health care practitioner, especially if your child has an autism spectrum disorder. There is a subset of children with autism that have metabolic disorders that may result in enzyme pathway problems. We recommend blood testing for amino acid levels as well as a metabolic workup (to the degree determined necessary by a health care practitioner) before using taurine.

TAURINE TOTAL DAILY GOAL DOSING

AGE	DOSE	FREQUENCY	TOTAL DAILY DOSE FROM ALL SOURCES
2 to 5	150 mg	1 or 2 times per day	300 mg
6 to 10	150 mg	2 times per day	300 mg
11 +	250 mg	2 times per day	500 mg

- Higher doses should be accomplished only under the guidance of a health care practitioner.
- Start at half of the lowest recommended dose and increase as tolerated.
- Watch for possible side effects and decrease the dose accordingly.
- If symptoms improve at lower than the goal dose, you may not need to continue to increase the dose.

TAURINE

Tests	Plasma amino acid testing
Supplement types	L-taurine
Side effects	Loose stools
Toxicity/symptoms of excess	Toxicity level not reported For those with unique metabolic dysfunctions, taurine may not be tolerated and should be avoided.
Sources	Meat, fish (especially shellfish)
Interactions	*Enhancers:* Taurine is synergistic with magnesium. Taurine may result in elevated lithium levels. *Antagonist:* In diabetes, increased intracellular accumulation of sorbitol can deplete taurine.

OTHER NUTRIENTS AND COFACTORS

■ *4.13 Carnitine*

Carnitine is synthesized in the body from the amino acids lysine and methionine. L-carnitine, a biologically active form of carnitine, helps the body turn fat into energy. It is made in the liver and kidneys and stored primarily in muscle. Because carnitine is necessary for the mitochondria to work optimally, low levels of carnitine can result in poor endurance, weak muscles (including weak cardiac muscles), low muscle tone, and fatigue.

Functions
- Generation of cellular energy via transporting long chain fatty acids into the mitochondria, for fatty acid oxidation
- Antioxidant
- Maintenance of muscle mass
- Maintenance of bone mass through increases in osteocalcin, a bone-building protein, which decreases with age.

Risks for deficiency
- Poor intake of red meat, the main dietary source of carnitine
- Deficiencies of nutrients required for the manufacture of carnitine: iron, B vitamins, lysine, methionine, and vitamin C
- Certain seizure medications (e.g., valproic acid), which can lower carnitine
- Genetic/metabolic disorders that reduce ability to make carnitine or are associated with low carnitine
- Periods of growth
- Pregnancy

Deficiency signs and symptoms
- Fatigue
- Poor endurance
- Weak muscles (including weak heart muscle)
- Low tone
- Poor glucose control

Carnitine and the Connection to ADHD and Autism

Low carnitine can occur in children with either ADHD or autism if their diets do not include sufficient carnitine sources, such as red meat. Children with autism are more likely to have carnitine deficiency due to the frequency of poor or restricted appetites. Some children with autism may have genetic difficulties in making carnitine or certain genetic disorders associated with low carnitine. Low carnitine can contribute to poor core energy metabolism, resulting in impaired muscle function. Food sources include red meat, chicken, fish, milk, and cheese.

Carnitine Supplements

There are two primary forms of carnitine supplements: L-carnitine and acetyl-L-carnitine. L-carnitine is recommended when treating general symptoms such as fatigue or poor endurance. Acetyl-L-carnitine may be more helpful for supporting brain function as it absorbs more readily and crosses the blood–brain barrier efficiently.

The D and DL forms of carnitine should be avoided. They are not functional and can cause serious problems. Lower doses of carnitine are used to treat

Carnitine

dietary causes of low carnitine while much higher doses may be needed to treat metabolic dysfunctions or inefficiencies.

Carnitine Dosing

Because of the possibility of an underlying rare disorder or potential problems from very low carnitine levels, L-carnitine supplementation is not recommended without blood testing. Supplementation should be accomplished only under the care of a health care practitioner. The practitioner can determine whether additional testing is indicated before carnitine use.

Dosing of carnitine is dependent on the cause of the low carnitine as well as the blood level.

Possible Side Effects

Some children with metabolic disorders may have a worsening of behavior on L-carnitine. This may either be a direct side effect of the supplement or a consequence of the body adjusting to increased energy and alertness from the benefits of carnitine. Loose stools are also possible. At high doses, carnitine can result in a fishy smell.

There are rare metabolic disorders (LCHAD, VLCAD) that can include cardiomyopathy (a weakening of the heart muscle). In these conditions, L-carnitine is potentially dangerous due to the possibility of causing abnormal heart rhythms. L-carnitine can also aggravate seizures in certain susceptible individuals. Cardiomyopathy can occur when carnitine levels are very low; hence, blood testing is important before L-carnitine is used.

■ 4.14 Coenzyme Q_{10} (CoQ$_{10}$, Ubiquinone/Ubiquinol)

Coenzyme Q_{10}, also known as ubiquinone or the more active form ubiquinol, is a fat-soluble compound primarily synthesized by the body and also consumed in the diet. CoQ$_{10}$ is found in virtually all cell membrane—hence the ubiquinone, because it is ubiquitous. Its primary function is to shuttle electrons through the electron transport chain into the mitochondria, the main energy-generating machinery of the cells. CoQ$_{10}$ is responsible for 95 percent of energy produced for the body. If there is deficiency in the enzyme or its function, the body experiences a "brown out" during which there is not sufficient energy to accomplish all of the body's functions. The result is fatigue, poor endurance, lethargy, and muscle weakness.

Our recommendations are focused on mitochondrial inefficiencies or dysfunctions, not the serious, life-threatening mitochondrial diseases. There is a subset of children with autism that have these lesser inefficiencies and dysfunctions that can be responsive to treatment.

Functions
- Shuttles electrons into the mitochondria to help generate ATP, the main energy molecule used by cells
- Gene expression

- Immunity
- Cardiovascular function
- Neurological function
- Potent antioxidant
- Blood-thinning capabilities

Risks for deficiency
- Medications (statins, beta-blockers, tricyclic antidepressants)
- Genetic metabolic disorders, e.g., those involving the electron transport chain/oxidative phosphorylation

CoQ_{10} Supplements

CoQ_{10} is fat soluble and best absorbed with fat in a meal. CoQ_{10} may be given as ubiquinone or as ubiquinol, the more active form with higher bioavailability.

CoQ_{10} TOTAL DAILY GOAL DOSING

AGE	DOSE	TOTAL DAILY DOSE FROM ALL SOURCES
2 to 5	25 to 50 mg	25 to 50 mg
6 to 10	50 to 75 mg	50 to 75 mg
11 +	100 mg	100 mg

- CoQ_{10} supplements are considered safe and no RDA or toxic dose has been identified.
- For higher doses, consult a health care practitioner.

■ 4.15 *Essential Omega-3 Fatty Acids*

There are two types of essential fatty acids: omega-3 and omega-6. Omega-3 includes the precursor source alpha-linolenic acid (ALA) and direct-sources eicosapentaenoic acid (EPA) and docosahexaenoic acid (DHA). Omega-6 includes the precursor linoleic acid and direct-source gamma-linolenic acid.

For optimal cell function, cell walls need to be flexible rather than rigid. Omega-3 fats are the most flexible fats. Approximately 60 percent of the dry weight of the brain is composed of fat including cholesterol and fatty acids. Omega-3 DHA is a critical structural component of the human brain, retina, and nerves. In the brain, omega-3 fatty acid deficiency can result in less than optimal transmission of messages.

Deficiency signs and symptoms
- Skin conditions: eczema, dermatitis, rashes, cradle cap, keratosis pilaris ("chicken skin")
- Developmental delays including poor motor development

- Language and communication delays (DHA)
- Impaired cognitive function (DHA)
- Mood and behavior disorders (DHA)
- ADHD symptoms (DHA)
- Vision dysfunction (DHA)
- Immune dysfunction
- Poor hair quality
- Hard earwax
- Excessive thirst
- Cracking or peeling nails

The ideal omega-6:omega-3 intake should be from 1:1 to 4:1. The Standard American diet is omega-6 excessive at 16:1. Excessive omega-6 and insufficient omega-3 intake increases inflammation, cardiovascular disease, cancer, and autoimmunity.

Omega-3 Fatty Acids Food Sources

The best food sources of omega-3 fatty acids are seafood. Those highest in mercury, PCBs, and other toxins include tomalley (crab mustard), farmed fish, trout, imported shrimp, and the large "steak" fish such as tuna, bluefish, swordfish, and shark. The safest choices include anchovies, sardines, domestic shrimp, rock-fish, and tilapia. For details, see the Environmental Working Group website, www.ewg.org, and the Environmental Defense Fund website, www.edf.org.

Omega-3 Fatty Acids Supplements

The best choices for omega-3 fatty acids are supplements containing preformed EPA and DHA to support brain, vision, and skin health. The skin benefits more from EPA, while DHA has greater impact on brain, vision, mood, behavior, and attention. Flaxseed oil is a source of the EPA and DHA precursor, ALA. The conversion of ALA to EPA and DHA is limited, especially in males, and flaxseed oil is therefore not a preferred source.

To achieve safe and adequate doses of omega-3 fatty acids, supplementation is required. It is critical that the supplement be as toxin-free as possible. Look for fish oil supplements that are pharmaceutical grade or have removed toxins via molecular distillation.

For vegetarians or those who are allergic to fish oils, DHA sources from algae are recommended. Neuromins is an algae-source version and is available in gel cap and liquid form. This form of omega-3 only contains DHA, not EPA.

Cod liver oils vary significantly in the amount of omega-3, vitamin A, and vitamin D. It is important to not exceed the total daily RDA for vitamin A if taking both cod liver oil and a multiple vitamin–mineral. Some specialty vitamin companies offer multiple vitamin–mineral combinations without vitamin A to help meet this need. Many omega-3 fish oils supplements have vitamin D_3 added, which may be sufficient to meet the recommendations for vitamin D_3.

In reality, the choice of fish oil often comes down to taste and palatability. We have listed several good quality options below.

EPA AND DHA DIRECT SOURCES

SUPPLEMENT COMPANY	SERVING SIZE	EPA	DHA	VITAMIN D₃*	VITAMIN A*	COMMENTS
Omega Swirl *Barlean's*	2 tsp	360 mg	360 mg	0	0	Tasty peach mango, or lemon smoothie
Omega Cure (unflavored) *Omega Cure*	1 tsp	500 mg	500 mg	0	0	No taste
ProOmega or Ultimate Omega† with or without D₃ *Nordic Naturals*	½ tsp	813 mg	563 mg	0 or 500 IU	0	Lemon flavor
ProOmega or Ultimate Omega soft gels† *Nordic Naturals*	1 soft gel	650 mg	450 mg	0 or 500 IU	0	Lemon flavor in the soft gel
Very Finest Fish Oil *Carlson Labs*	1 tsp	800 mg	500 mg	0	0	Lemon flavor
Coromega Squeeze† with or without D₃ *Coromega*	1 pkt	350 mg	230 mg	0 or 1,000 IU	0	Many flavors Contains egg Avoid orange, which contains vanillin
Norwegian Cod Liver Oil† with A and D₃ *Carlson Labs*	1 tsp	400 mg	500 mg	400 IU	850 IU	Lemon flavor
Cod Liver Oil† with or without A and D₃ *Kirkman Labs*	½ tsp	250 mg	250 mg	0 or 250 IU	0 or 2,500 IU	Flavored or unflavored
Baby's DHA (and EPA)† *Nordic Naturals*	4 ml	328 mg	480 mg	250 IU	340 to 1,200 IU	
Flaxseed Oil *Barlean's, Spectrum Support*	1 tsp	0	0	0	0	2,000 mg ALA precursor
Neuromins DHA caps†† *Source Naturals, Pure Encaps*	1 soft gel	0	200 mg	0	0	Vegetarian source
Neuromins DHA liquid†† *Source Naturals, Pure Encaps*	1 ml	0	280 mg	0	0	Vegetarian source
ProDHA 1,000 soft gels†† *Nordic Naturals*	1 soft gel	90 mg	450 mg	0	0	Lemon flavor in the soft gel
Super DHA Liquid *Genestra*	½ tsp	130 mg	600 mg	0	0	Oil of orange flavor

*Include the amount of vitamin A and vitamin D as part of the total daily dose
†Vitamins A and D content of omega-3 oils
††DHA-only sources

Omega-3 Fatty Acids

- DHA is more specific to development and retina, cognition, and language.
- For other omega-3 deficiency symptoms, EPA should be taken as well. Pay attention to the serving size, particularly for soft gels. The total amount of DHA listed may be for a serving size of more than one soft gel.
- The milligram amounts listed above were accurate at the time of writing of this book. As product compositions may change, always check the labels of products.
- Refrigerating the oils helps prolong shelf life and also improves palatability.

Omega-3 Fatty Acids Dosing

Supplements come with different ratios of EPA and DHA. The minimum amount of DHA recommended for school-age children is 400 mg. However, recent research shows that children with autism may require higher dosing. We recommend supplements that combine both EPA and DHA, even though dosing focuses on the DHA levels as those with ADHD or autism typically have significant needs for the DHA.

OMEGA-3 EPA AND DHA TOTAL DAILY GOAL DOSING

AGE	EPA	DHA	FREQUENCY
2 to 5	200 to 400 mg	200 to 400 mg	Daily with food
6 to 10	500 to 650 mg	400 to 500 mg	Daily with food
11 +	500 to 800 mg	500 to 650 mg	Daily with food

Higher doses of the omega-3 fatty acids may be indicated for your child; however, dosing should be determined by a health care practitioner.

FLAXSEED OIL TOTAL DAILY GOAL DOSING

AGE	DOSE	FREQUENCY
2 to 5	1 tsp	1 time per day with food
6 to 10	1 tsp	1 or 2 times per day with food
11 +	1 tsp	2 or 3 times per day with food

Flaxseed oil capsules/soft gels contain a very low dose of flaxseed. Use of liquid is recommended for better dosing.

Possible Side Effects

Side effects to fish oils are unusual. Some fish oils contain ingredients to which children with food sensitivities may react. For example, Coromega contains egg and some fish oils contain soy.

Some children may develop loose stools from fish oils. At high doses, fish oils can affect platelet function and may result in easy bruising. This is uncommon.

A small number of children become irritable when starting cod liver oil. We theorize this may be related to changes in vision, analogous to the transiently irritating experience of adjusting to stronger or different eyeglass prescriptions. We therefore recommend starting with half the recommended dose for one week and then increasing to the full dose.

Additional Information

For vitamin A content, make sure that the total from cod liver oil, the multiple vitamin–mineral supplement, and additional vitamin A do not exceed the following doses:

VITAMIN A TOTAL DAILY GOAL DOSING

AGE	DAILY DOSE
2 to 3	1,250 IU
4 to 5	1,250 to 2,500 IU
6 to 10	2,500 to 3,500 IU
11 +	3,500 to 5,000 IU

We recommend using a fish oil without vitamin A as your main source of omega-3 fatty acids. For children who require additional vitamin A (e.g., for eye contact, skin, oxidative stress treatment, etc.), vitamin A may be given from a separate supplement source.

Because omega-3 fatty acids can affect platelet function (relevant to blood clotting), it is advisable to stop fish oils before elective surgeries or procedures. The usual recommendation is to stop for three to five days before the procedure and for two to five days after, depending on the type of surgery; check with your physician or dentist to determine whether there is a more specific recommendation for your child.

▪ 4.16 Probiotics

Probiotics are beneficial live microorganisms called the microbiome found in the intestinal tract. There are more than 100 trillion good bacteria in the body with 500 to 1,000 different species (forty to fifty of which are main species) in the human gut.

Functions

- Immune support (70 percent of total body immunity is located in the intestinal mucosal tissues, "fed" by good flora)
- Production of nutrients that can be depleted by antibiotic use, such as biotin, vitamin K, and B vitamins

Probiotics

- Fermentation of dietary fiber and "prebiotic" indigestible complex carbohydrates such as inulin and fructo-oligosaccharides to produce healthy, short chain fatty acids for digestive health and immunity. Prebiotics nourish the growth of probiotics.
- Reduction of inflammation
- Inhibition of the growth of harmful bacteria
- Improved digestion and nutrient absorption
- Removal of toxins
- Reduction in allergies and skin conditions

Risks for deficiency
- Antibiotic use
- Poor dietary fiber intake

Conditions that may improve with probiotic use
- Diarrhea
- Constipation
- Peristalsis, bowel transit time
- Intestinal infections caused by antibiotics (yeast/*Candida, C. difficile*)
- Rotavirus incidence
- Digestive tract inflammation (gastritis, duodenitis, colitis)
- Systemic (total body) inflammation
- Eczema
- Allergies
- Asthma

The use of probiotics in pregnancy and lactation significantly reduces the risk for infant asthma, allergy, and eczema for up to two years.

Food sources
- Beneficial bacteria: fermented foods such as yogurts, kefir, buttermilk, fermented vegetables, sauerkraut, tempeh, miso, coconut kefir, and kimchi
- Prebiotics: fruits, legumes, some vegetables, and whole grains

Probiotics and the Connection to ADHD and Autism

Imbalanced intestinal bacteria and yeast overgrowth are conditions commonly seen in children with autism and to a somewhat lesser degree in children with ADHD. Antibiotic use can lead to these imbalances by killing beneficial bacteria in the intestine. When bacteria are present in suboptimal numbers, yeast and other problematic bacteria can inappropriately flourish. Resulting problems can include both physical symptoms (e.g., diaper rashes, loose stools, gas) and behavioral symptoms (e.g., inattention, silly giggling, etc.). Refer to section 2.18 Yeast Overgrowth. Probiotics help restore appropriate balance of bacteria in the intestine.

Probiotic Supplements

There are numerous choices in probiotics, with an extremely wide range of strengths and types of bacteria.

- May be in single strain to multistrain cultures (*Lactobacillus, Bifidobacterium, Streptococcus, Saccharomyces*)
- Should contain live strains, be stored in freezers prior to use, be shipped on ice, and be stored in the refrigerator during use
- Should be hypoallergenic (no milk, casein, gluten, soy, corn, or artificial additives)

Types of supplements

- *Bifidus infantis* or bifido complexes (for infants)
- *Lactobacillus acidophilus*
- *Lactobacillus/Bifidus* combinations
- Expanded combinations with multiple strains
- *Saccharomyces boulardii* (a "beneficial" yeast)

PROBIOTIC TYPES AND FUNCTIONS

TYPE OF PROBIOTIC	INFORMATION	FUNCTIONS
Bifidobacterium	Found primarily in the colon *Bifidus infantis* (lactis)—best for infants	Treats colic, cradle cap, eczema, allergies Anti-inflammatory
Lactobacillus	Found primarily in the small intestine	GI health Improved digestion
Streptococcus thermophilus	Helpful, transient good bacteria	Enhances production of bifidobacteria
Saccharomyces boulardii	Friendly yeast Not to be taken with antifungal medications	Enhances secretory IgA Controls *Candida albicans* (yeast), diarrhea, *Clostridium difficile*

Source: Digestive Wellness for Children *by Elizabeth Lipski.*

- For infants and those with sensitive digestive tracts, try single supplements of *Bifidus* to start and then expand to *Lactobacillus*.
- For those who are intolerant to disaccharides and use the Specific Carbohydrate Diet (SCD, see page 239), avoid prebiotics such as inulin and oligosaccharides.
- Consider rotating supplements to expand the variety of bacteria available.

Probiotics

PROBIOTIC PRODUCTS

HYPOALLERGENIC PROBIOTICS COMPANY	TYPE	CFUS PER DOSE	COMMENTS
Ultra Bifidus Dairy Free made by *Metagenics*	*Bifido infantis* (B. lactis)	15 billion per ½ tsp	Best for infants
Bifido Complex Advanced Inulin Free made by *Kirkman Labs*	*Bifidobacterium lactis, B. bifidum, B. longum, B. breve*	15 billion per capsule	Best for infants to age 2 Specific Carbohydrate Diet (SCD) compliant
Lactobacillus acidophilus made by *Kirkman Labs* and *Klaire Labs*	One strain only	3 billion per capsule	SCD compliant (no disaccharides)
Ther-Biotic Infant Formula with Inulin made by *Klaire Labs*	*Lactobacillus* and *Bifidobacterium* 10 mixed strains	10 billion per ¼ tsp	Broad spectrum support for infant GI tract Good for formula-fed babies or those born by C section
Lactobacillus Duo made by *Kirkman Labs*	*L. rhamnosus* L. plantarum	30 billion per capsule	Improves health of intestinal cells Reduced respiratory infections in children Antimicrobial SCD compliant
Pro-Bio Gold with Inulin made by *Kirkman Labs* Pro-Bio Inulin Free made by *Kirkman Labs* Pro-Bio Chewable Wafer made by *Kirkman Labs*	*Lactobacillus* and *Bifidobacterium* 6 mixed strains	20 billion per capsule 20 billion per wafer	Comprehensive broad spectrum for small and large intestine Wafer contains xylitol, which reduces dental decay
Pro-5 (5 strains) made by *Klaire Labs* Ther-Biotic Children's Chewable (4 strains) made by *Klaire Labs*	*Lactobacillus* and *Bifidobacterium* mixed strains	25 billion per capsule 25 billion per wafer	Comprehensive broad spectrum Wafer contains xylitol, which reduces dental decay
S. boulardii made by *Kirkman Labs,* *Klaire Labs*	*S. boulardii*	3 billion CFUs	"Beneficial" yeast

• CFUs stands for Colony Forming Units

PROBIOTIC TOTAL DAILY GOAL DOSING

AGE	DOSE IN CFUS	FREQUENCY TAKE WITH FOOD
1 to 2	1 to 5 billion	Begin with single *Bifidobacterium* product. Expand to mixed cultures for infants, especially if formula fed.
3 to 5	5 to 10 billion	In two divided doses
6 to 10	10 to 20 billion	In two divided doses
11 +	10 to 50 billion	In two divided doses

- Start low and increase slowly to avoid die-off side effects.
- For products with 5 to 10 billion bacteria, start with one-quarter to one-half capsule once daily and increase by one-quarter to one-half capsule every two to three days until on goal dose or die-off symptoms develop.
- For higher dose probiotics, start with one-quarter capsule and increase by one-quarter capsule every two to three days.
- Probiotics are best taken with cool, mild-temperature food and can also be taken on an empty stomach.
- If taking antibiotics, wait at least one hour before giving probiotics.
- Consult with a practitioner for use of higher doses of probiotics.

Possible Side Effects
When there are insufficient good bacteria in the intestine, other organisms such as yeast or *Clostridia* bacteria can overgrow. When good bacteria are reintroduced, yeast and *Clostridia* organisms can die and release toxins, which if not adequately excreted, can be absorbed into the bloodstream and cause behavioral side effects, commonly referred to as "die-off" effects.

The most common initial side effect is irritability. With more significant die-off, overall behavior can worsen (e.g., temper tantrums, behavioral regression). For this reason, it is important for the child to have daily stools when on probiotics in order to adequately excrete toxins. Starting with a low dose of probiotic and increasing slowly allows you to detect side effects at their initial stages so that probiotic dosing can be decreased to a tolerable level.

Tests
Stool cultures for types and amounts of beneficial bacteria, pathogenic/problematic bacteria, and yeast can be performed through specialty labs (such as Doctors Data, Metametrix, Genova Diagnostics, Great Plains, etc.). Stool testing from standard laboratories does not provide this type of detailed testing. Urine testing through specialized laboratories can identify the metabolites (by-products) produced by bacteria, yeast, parasites, and other pathogens.

■ *4.17 Digestive Enzymes*
Digestive enzymes can be used as part of the treatment for food sensitivities and intolerances, including casein, gluten, and soy, the most commonly problematic food proteins in ADHD and autism.

A full discussion of food sensitivities and intolerances in ADHD and autism is beyond the scope of this book. Refer to our first book, *The Kid-Friendly ADHD & Autism Cookbook*, for detailed information. In short, food proteins, particularly those from milk (casein) and wheat (gluten), may be incompletely digested to peptides and may enter the bloodstream from the intestine via an abnormally permeable intestinal lining ("leaky gut"). These partially digested proteins can then potentially cross the blood–brain barrier and enter the brain where they can negatively affect brain function by several mechanisms:

Digestive Enzymes

- Blocking neurotransmitter messages
- Creating opiate-like doping effects from gluten (gliadorphin) and milk casein (casomorphin)
- Triggering brain inflammation

Effects may occur within an hour of consumption or be delayed up to seventy-two hours.

There are two main treatment strategies for treating food intolerances and the opiate-like effect:

1. Gluten-Free Casein-Free Soy-Free (GFCFSF) Diet—Elimination Trial: the "gold standard" for treatment
   - The most common problem food proteins are gluten, milk casein, and soy.
   - Your child's body is the best test. Eliminate the food(s) to see whether behavior improves and reintroduce or challenge the body to see whether behavior worsens.
2. Digestive enzymes, including dipeptidyl peptidase-IV (DPP-IV)
   - More efficiently digest gluten, casein, soy, and other food proteins, carbohydrates, and fats.
   - Reduce the opioid load due to insufficient DPP-IV enzyme function; this can also "mimic" the diet.

Sometimes it is not possible to remove foods from the diet immediately. The opioid effect from gluten and milk casein can result in an addiction to the food sources and cause limitation of other foods. In these picky eaters, removing milk products and/or wheat and gluten eliminates most of their foods. It can be more feasible to start with digestive enzymes to reduce the opioid load, which can also partially "mimic" an elimination diet. During this time, gluten-free and casein-free foods can be introduced. While there is variance among individuals, for some children, digestive enzymes can be about 50 percent as effective as an elimination diet. For others, diet compliance must be 100 percent. Enzyme use is not an equivalent substitute for an elimination diet.

Digestive enzymes may support general digestion or may be specific to digesting opiate-like peptides. Some supplements combine both types. See the chart below.

DIGESTIVE ENZYME INDICATORS

TYPE OF DIGESTIVE ENZYMES	SYMPTOMS THAT INDICATE A NEED FOR THE ENZYMES
General digestive enzymes *Digest protein (protease), sugars (disaccharidases), starches (cellulase), and fats (lipase)*	Undigested food in stool, foul smell to stools Oily, light-colored, or foamy stools Bloating, intestinal gas
DPP-IV (Dipeptidyl peptidase-IV) *Digests opioid peptides: gliadorphin from gluten and casomorphin from casein*	Consumption of gluten and/or milk casein results in brain fog, irritability

DIGESTIVE ENZYME SUPPLEMENTS

DIGESTIVE ENZYMES	FUNCTION	PRODUCTS
DPP-IV	Digests the opioid peptides from poor digestion of gluten, milk casein, and possibly soy.	DPP-IV Forte, made by *Kirkman Labs* Peptizyde, made by *Houston Enzymes*
Combination General and DPP-IV	Digests proteins, fats, carbohydrates, and opioid peptides	EnZym-Complete/DPP-IV, made by *Kirkman Labs* TriEnza (includes No-Fenol), made by *Houston Enzymes*

DIPEPTIDYL PEPTIDASE-IV SINGULARLY OR WITH OTHER ENZYMES— TOTAL DAILY GOAL DOSING

AGE	DOSE	FREQUENCY
2 to 5	½ capsule	3 times per day with meals, one additional dose with snack
6 to 10	1 capsule	3 times per day with meals, one additional dose with snack
11 +	1 to 2 capsules	3 times per day with meals, one additional dose with snack

- Start with one-half capsule once daily at breakfast, gradually increasing by one-half capsule every three days, until on goal dose.
- One additional dose may be used during the day for a snack that contains offending foods, given at least an hour away from other enzyme doses.
- Withdrawal symptoms can occur, resulting in temporary irritability and worsened behavior.
- Once the enzymes are added to food or liquid, they become activated. They cannot be added to food or liquid and used at a later time.
- If your child attends school, you will need a medication form to be given the enzyme right before lunch.
- Enzymes are best taken at the beginning of the meal or snack. If the dose is delayed, enzymes can be given during the meal and up to one hour after (the length of time food takes to clear the stomach).
- The enzyme capsule can be swallowed or opened and the powder mixed into food or liquid.

Possible Side Effects

Some children have "withdrawal" symptoms with removal of opioid foods or use of digestive enzymes that digest the opioids. This often manifests as irritability or worsened behavior. Some children may also have an increased craving for the foods that have been removed. Rarely, diarrhea can occur.

The main contraindication to taking digestive enzymes is stomach irritation. This is unusual in children. However, if your child has significant gastrointestinal symptoms, including significant reflux symptoms, discuss enzyme use with your child's physician.

Digestive Enzymes

Combination Digestive Enzymes

Some children who have opioid problems may also have disaccharidase deficiency and benefit from the SCD diet and/or have phenol sulfotransferase deficiency and benefit from the low phenol diet. For these individuals, there are enzymes applicable to each situation.

COMPLETE DIGESTIVE ENZYME TOTAL DAILY GOAL DOSING

PRODUCT COMPANY	DESCRIPTIONS	SCD- AND GFCF-COMPLIANT	AGE	PER MEAL
ProZymes made by *GI ProHealth*	Combination enzymes: general digestion, DPP-IV, disaccharidases	Yes	2 to 5 6 to 10 11 +	½ to 1 capsule 1 capsule 2 capsules
Maximum Spectrum EnzymComplete DPP-IV Fruit Free with Isogest made by *Kirkman Labs*	Combination enzymes: general digestion, DPP-IV, disaccharidases	Yes	2 to 5 6 to 10 11 +	½ to 1 capsule 1 capsule 2 capsules
TriEnza made by *Houston Enzymes*	Combination enzymes: general digestion, DPP-IV, disaccharidases, phenolic	Yes	2 to 5 6 to 10 11 +	½ to 1 capsule 1 capsule 1 to 2 capsules

CHAPTER 5

Avoiding Traffic Accidents and Traffic Jams: Toxic Metals and Nutrient/ Medication/Herb/Food Interactions

Ubiquitous toxic metal exposures and problematic medication–nutrient interactions have the ability to significantly impair nutritional status and cellular enzyme functions. Among the most vulnerable to these negative effects are children with autism and to a lesser degree, those with ADHD, who have nutrient deficiencies and weaknesses in their detoxification systems.

■ 5.1 Toxic Metals

Toxic metals form poisonous soluble compounds and have no beneficial biological role in the human body. They may take the place of an essential element in the body. This chapter covers the common toxic metals: aluminum, arsenic, cadmium, lead, and mercury.

The body uses nutrients such as sulfur, zinc, selenium, and calcium to rid toxic metals such as mercury, cadmium, lead, and others. When the protective nutrients are deficient, toxic metals can accumulate in the body, eventually damaging normal body processes and eliciting symptoms. For example, mercury, cadmium, and lead can interfere with zinc bioavailability and function resulting in zinc deficiency symptoms such as picky appetite, increased infections, low muscle tone, skin conditions, and more.

Toxic Metals and the Connection to ADHD and Autism

If one or more detoxification systems are weak, as is more often seen in children with autism, the body is less able to handle toxic exposures. Individuals with autism and ADHD can have factors that render them more susceptible to toxic exposures, including poor digestion, impaired absorption, nutrient deficiencies, and inefficiencies in pathways supporting detoxification (e.g., methylation and sulfation).

Toxic Metal Sources

Common sources of toxic metals include industrial air and water contamination in addition to the following more specific sources:

- Aluminum: aluminum cans and cookware, food additives, processed foods, antacids, and antiperspirants.
- Arsenic: car batteries, herbicides, treated wood, seafood, and poultry.
- Cadmium: cigarettes, foods, plastics, and hazardous waste sites.
- Lead: lead paint, specific imported dishes and toys, pollution, and storage batteries.
- Mercury: dental amalgams; thimerosal in medications and some vaccines; and from consumption of large steak fish, such as tuna, bluefish, swordfish, and mackerel.

Toxic metals deplete nutrients that are needed or "spent" in order to rid the body of the toxins. Exposure to and accumulation of toxic metals significantly increases the risk for developmental delays, cognitive deficits, organ damage, neurological disorders including seizures, nutrient depletion, and anemia. The severity of the damage depends upon the number and levels of toxic exposures, the length of time exposed, and the individual's detoxification integrity.

Core Nutrients in Toxic Metal Removal

Because nutrients are critical to the processes that metabolize and remove toxins, they are an important component of the treatment methods for toxicity. Critical minerals include zinc, selenium, magnesium, calcium, and iron. The important vitamins are vitamins A, C, D, and the complex of B vitamins. The sulfur-bearing nutrients so critical to toxin removal include glutathione, N-acetyl cysteine, and alpha-lipoic acid, which generates glutathione. Epsom salt (magnesium sulfate) baths provide absorbable sulfate.

Testing for Toxic Metals

Although hair analysis is a screening tool for toxic exposures, more specific testing includes whole blood toxic metal analysis and porphyrin urine evaluation. There are also metabolic markers that can indicate possible toxic metal exposures including significantly low ferritin, zinc, and/or selenium, which are difficult to resolve.

Any level of a toxic metal is a problem. The higher the exposure, the greater and more significant the damage.

■ 5.2 *Medication/Nutrient/Herb Interactions*

Medication reactions depend upon the status of the individual's digestive system, detoxification ability, immune status, drug-metabolizing capability, and intake of foods, nutrients, herbs, and other medications, which can interact with each other.

When there is decreased or increased activity in one or more of the "drug metabolizing" cytochrome P450 enzymes, the body can produce unique reactions to certain medications that are metabolized by those enzymes. The abnormal reactions can include the following:

- Decreased metabolism/clearing resulting in an exaggerated response to a normal or low dose of a medication and a higher than expected medication blood level.
- Increased metabolism/clearing resulting in little to no effect from a normal or high dose of a medication and lower than expected medication blood level.

"Idiopathic" is the medical term for reactions for which there "appear" to be no explanation. For many such reactions, the explanation lies in understanding the metabolism of the medications and the competency of the individual's enzymes and nutritional status.

The Grapefruit/Citrus Juice Effect

One of the best-known food–medication interactions is "the grapefruit juice effect." The juice components responsible are called furanocoumarins. These irreversibly inhibit the cytochrome P450(CYP) 3A4 enzymes in the intestinal wall up to seventy-two hours after grapefruit consumption. The inhibition impairs the enzymes' ability to clear the medication resulting in a higher-than-expected level of medication circulating in the blood, potentially increasing the medication's toxic effects.

MEDICATION–NUTRIENT INTERACTIONS

MEDICATION	RESULTING NUTRIENT DEFICIENCIES	INFORMATION
Antacids H2 receptor antagonist proton pump inhibitors (PPIs) Prilosec Prevacid	B vitamins Minerals Protein Amino acids	Lower gastric pH from antacids increases the risk for many deficiencies because of impaired digestion and/or absorption. If reflux is the issue, it is important to determine underlying possible causes, including food reactions/intolerances (especially milk, gluten, and soy) and medical conditions.
Antacids Calcium-containing: Carbonate Tums Mylanta	Magnesium Phosphorus Copper Manganese Potassium Zinc Protein Folate	Increased risk for kidney stones due to magnesium depletion Avoid taking these antacids within 2 hours of consuming: • Minerals • High-phytate foods (beans, nuts) • High-oxalate foods (spinach, peanut butter, chocolate) • High-fiber foods Avoid in hypercalcemia (high blood calcium)
Antibiotics Broad-spectrum augmentin	Biotin Vitamins: B complex, C, K	Deplete good flora and vitamins they produce (biotin, vitamin K) Increased risk for yeast overgrowth

MEDICATION	RESULTING NUTRIENT DEFICIENCIES	INFORMATION
Antibiotics Tetracycline Doxycycline	Vitamins: B complex, C Calcium Magnesium Manganese Zinc	Deplete good flora and vitamins they produce (biotin, vitamin K) Increased risk for yeast overgrowth Chelate (bind to) minerals and interfere with absorption Elevated liver enzymes and reduced kidney function Avoid taking these antibiotics: • 1 hour before to 2 hours after food or milk • Within 2 hours of minerals • With vitamin A • With St. John's wort Avoid in: • Pregnancy • Children ≤ 8 years (will cause permanent damage to tooth enamel)
Antibiotics Cephalosporins	Vitamins: B complex Biotin	Deplete good flora and vitamins they produce (biotin, vitamin K) Increased risk for yeast overgrowth Inhibit a specific liver enzyme that can lead to vitamin K deficiency, liver damage, and reduced kidney function
Antibiotics Bactrim	Vitamins: B complex especially folate Biotin K	Deplete good flora and vitamins they produce (biotin, vitamin K) Increased risk for yeast overgrowth from depletion of good flora Possible respiratory damage in immune-compromised patients Elevated liver enzymes and reduced kidney function Avoid taking with St. John's wort
Antifungal Ketoconazole	Vitamin D	Impairs synthesis of vitamin D Risk for low white blood cell count and high triglycerides Negative effect on liver
Antifungal Nystatin	None known	Gastrointestinal effect only (not absorbed) Can cause GI distress, diarrhea
Antihistamines	None known	Avoid grapefruit juice up to 72 hours before taking Allegra, Singulair No grapefruit effect with Zyrtec or Benadryl
Antiseizure Phenytoin (Dilantin) Carbamazepine (Tegretol, Carbetrol) Primidone	Vitamins: folate, B_{12}, D, E Biotin Calcium	Long-term use increases risk for folate and B_{12} deficiency, anemia, and methylation defects Biotin depletion increases risk for dysbiosis (imbalanced intestinal bacteria) Avoid star fruit and pomegranate juice Phenytoin: avoid St. John's wort Primidone: avoid St. John's wort and quinine Carbamazepine: avoid grapefruit juice up to 72 hours before dose
Laxative and *Antidiarrhea* FiberCon Citrucel	Minerals	Bulk forming, binds with minerals, which can reduce their absorption Avoid taking within 2 hours of minerals
Laxatives *Softeners* Docusates Bisacodyl	Potassium Magnesium	Stomach discomfort Nausea

MEDICATION	RESULTING NUTRIENT DEFICIENCIES	INFORMATION
Laxatives Hyperosmotics (Glycolax, MiraLAX, Lactulose)	Folate Minerals	Poor absorption of nutrients Dehydration with long-term use Lactulose helps the body excrete ammonia and can increase glucose in diabetics
Laxatives Mineral oil	Fat-soluble vitamins Fatty acids Calcium Phosphorus Potassium	Poor absorption of nutrients Dehydration with long-term use Best to avoid
Laxatives Stimulants Senokot Dulcolax	Potassium Sodium	Melanosis coli (dark pigment on the colon) Does not resolve the underlying potential causes of constipation: dehydration or inadequate fiber, magnesium, and/or choline
Psychiatric for ADHD Intuniv/Tenex Clonidine	None known	Avoid licorice, grapefruit (Intuniv/Tenex)
Psychiatric SSRIs (Prozac, Zoloft, Celexa)	B vitamin complex Coenzyme Q_{10} Calcium Magnesium	Take with food Avoid: grapefruit juice, St, John's wort, tryptophan, 5-HTP Elevated liver enzymes Can increase cholesterol and triglycerides Can cause glucose fluctuations in diabetics Can deplete melatonin Folate enhances SSRI action
Psychiatric Neuroleptics Risperdal	Potassium Sodium	Elevated liver enzymes Low hemoglobin, hematocrit Increases uric acid, triglycerides, glucose Melatonin can reduce movement disorder side effects
Psychiatric Stimulants (Ritalin, Focalin, Concerta, Vyvanse, Adderall)	Vitamin B_{12} Vitamin C Potassium	Avoid St. John's wort and caffeine Elevated liver enzymes
Psychiatric Tricyclics	Coenzyme Q_{10} Vitamin B_2	Inhibit the production of CoQ_{10} Inhibit the absorption of B_2 Avoid taking with fiber, caffeine Clomiprimine: avoid grapefruit juice and St. John's wort Negative effect on liver, blood glucose (high and low)

Sources:
- "Interactions of Drugs, Nutritional Supplements and Dietary Components." In Lord RS & Bralley JA (Eds.). *Laboratory Evaluations for Integrative and Functional Medicine*, 2nd ed.; Appendix C
- *Food-Medication Interactions*, 17th ed. www.foodmedinteractions.com
- *Herb-Drug Interaction Handbook*, 3rd ed.
- University of Maryland Medical Center Complementary and Alternative Medicine Index, www.umm.edu/altmed

Medication/Nutrient/Herb/Food Interactions

CHAPTER 6

The Right Fuel: An Overview of Special Diets

There are many special diets that can be helpful for children with ADHD or autism. A detailed discussion of these diets is beyond the scope of this book, although we have provided a brief description of each diet along with helpful resources.

■ 6.1 Gluten-, Casein-, and Soy-Free (GFCSF) Diet

The GFCFSF diet involves the elimination of gluten, casein, and soy. Gluten is the main protein in wheat, oat, barley, rye, spelt, and Kamut. Casein is the main protein in animal milk products. Soy includes edamame, miso, natto, tamari, tempeh, tofu, and any products from soy. This is the most commonly utilized diet in the treatment of autism and may also benefit children with ADHD and other behavioral or developmental challenges.

Casein, gluten, and soy may be incompletely digested to peptides and may enter the bloodstream from the intestine via an abnormally permeable intestinal lining (referred to as "leaky gut"). These partially digested protein peptides can potentially cross the blood–brain barrier, negatively affecting brain function, and contributing to mood and behavior by blocking neurotransmitter messages, causing an opiate-like doping effect from gluten and milk casein, and/or triggering brain inflammation.

When gluten and milk casein are incompletely digested because of deficiency or inefficiency of the dipeptidyl peptidase-IV (DPP-IV) enzyme, the opiate-like peptides called gliadorphin from gluten and casomorphin from casein become available for absorption and can cross into the brain.

The best indicators for trying the GFCFSF diet include cravings for the opioid food sources, and limited appetite for other foods. The most common changes after starting the diet include improved eye contact, attention, language, and stool quality, and reduced or resolved self-stimulating behavior and self-injury. In addition to diet restrictions, treatment can also include use of the DPP-IV digestive enzymes, which are helpful in weaning onto the diet and for hidden exposures to gluten and/or casein.

Helpful resources
- *The Kid-Friendly ADHD & Autism Cookbook* by the authors
- *Special Diets for Special Kids Volumes 1 and 2 Combined* by Lisa Lewis
- *Cooking to Heal* by Julie Matthews
- The GFCF Diet Intervention—Autism Diet, www.gfcfdiet.com

■ 6.2 Low Phenol/Salicylate (Feingold) Diet

Phenols and salicylates are naturally occurring chemicals found in a number of foods, particularly fruits and vegetables such as apples, red grapes, and tomatoes. They can also be found in a variety of artificial food additives. The enzyme, phenol sulfotransferase (PST), uses sulfate to metabolize phenols. When PST and/or sulfate are deficient, phenols fail to be metabolized well and reactions occur. A subset of children, especially those with autism, do not have adequate levels of sulfate. Artificial food additives, colorings, flavorings, and pesticides are the most significant load on the PST system.

The best indicators for trying the diet are the following symptoms, which appear especially after consumption of foods or medications with artificial ingredients, and/or phenol foods: red cheeks and ears, silly behavior, aggression, hyperactivity, night sweats, and craving for phenols and salicylates.

The Failsafe diet (Free of Additives, Low in Salicylates, Amines, and Flavor Enhancers) expands upon the low phenol diet. Helpful resources:
- See section 2.15 Silly Behavior and Inappropriate Giggling/Laughing
- Feingold diet:
  - *Why Can't My Child Behave?* by Jane Hersey
  - www.feingold.org
- Failsafe diet:
  - *Fed Up* by Sue Dengate
  - www.failsafediet.wordpress.com

■ 6.3 Specific Carbohydrate Diet (SCD) and Gut and Psychology Syndrome (GAPS) Diet

The SCD addresses problems with the digestion of double-sugar disaccharides (lactose, sucrose, maltose, and isomaltose) found in sugar, grains, starches, beans, and most milk products. The diet is indicated when there is persistence of digestive problems (gas, diarrhea, and yeast overgrowth), especially when starchy disaccharide foods are consumed. This is more likely in those with damaged intestines and inadequate disaccharidase enzymes.

SCD is based on the principle that simple monosaccharides (fructose, glucose, and galactose) found in fruits, nonstarch vegetables, and honey require minimal digestion, are well absorbed, and leave no undigested residues. The residues of the undigested double sugars become food for intestinal "bad bugs" and yeast resulting in a "cesspool" within the gut. This leads to digestive distress including gas, bloating, cramps, abnormal stools, constipation, and diarrhea. The result is poor absorption of nutrients. Disaccharide intolerance is common in many bowel conditions including Crohn's disease, colitis, inflammatory bowel conditions, and irritable bowel syndrome. The GAPS diet further expands on this treatment protocol.

Beyond dietary restrictions, treatment usually includes supplementing with disaccharidase enzymes. Helpful resources:
- *Breaking the Vicious Cycle* by Elaine Gottschall
- www.breakingtheviciouscycle.info
- www.scdiet.com
- www.gapsdiet.com

■ 6.4 Anti-Yeast/Anti-Candida Diet and the Body Ecology Diet (BED)

These diets are helpful for individuals who have chronic intestinal yeast overgrowth that is not adequately treated by probiotics and antifungal medications or herbs. Anti-yeast diets avoid foods that feed yeast overgrowth such as sugars, yeast, starches, fruit juices, refined grains, and processed meats. The Body Ecology Diet addresses yeast overgrowth but also includes other dietary principles including those from macrobiotic, raw food, blood type, and Weston A. Price diets. Beyond dietary restrictions and food combining, treatments usually include probiotics and fermented foods and can expand to antifungal herbs and medications. Helpful resources:
- Section 2.18 Yeast Overgrowth
- *The Yeast Connection* by William Crook, M.D., www.yeastconnection.com
- *The Body Ecology Diet* by Donna Gates, www.bodyecology.com

■ 6.5 Low Oxalate Diet (LOD)

Oxalates are abundant in seeds and nuts and are present in many plants and fruits. Excess oxalates can also occur from intestinal oxalate-forming fungi and insufficient good flora to bind them for removal. Oxalates can cause digestive pain and when absorbed via a "leaky gut" can elicit systemic pain and kidney stones. Deficiencies of vitamin B_6 and magnesium can increase oxalate levels.

A low oxalate diet can be very difficult to follow; we do not recommend it as a first-line dietary intervention. We do recommend the use of probiotics and supplementation with vitamin B_6 and magnesium, which help clear oxalates from the body. Helpful resource:
- www.lowoxalate.info

References

Books
Baker, Sidney M., Jon Pangborn, and Bernard Rimland. 2005. *Autism: Effective Biomedical Treatments*. San Diego: Autism Research Institute.

Baker, Sidney M. and Jon Pangborn. 2007. *Supplement—Autism: Effective Biomedical Treatments*. San Diego: Autism Research Institute.

Bock, Kenneth, and Cameron Stauth. 2008. *Healing the New Childhood Epidemics*. New York: Ballantine.

Devlin, Thomas M., ed. 2006. *Textbook of Biochemistry with Clinical Correlations*, 6th ed. Hoboken: Wiley-Liss.

Gropper, Sareen S., Jack L. Smith, and James L. Groff. 2009. *Advanced Nutrition and Human Metabolism*, 5th ed. Stamford: Wadsworth.

Herbert, Martha, and Karen Weintraub. 2012. *The Autism Revolution: Whole-Body Strategies for Making Life All It Can Be*. New York: Ballantine.

Jepson, Bryan, Katie Wright, and Jane Johnson. 2007. *Changing the Course of Autism*. Boulder: Sensient.

Kohlstadt, Ingrid, ed. 2009. *Food and Nutrients in Disease Management*. Boca Raton: CRC Press.

Lord, Richard S., and J. Alexander Bralley. 2008. *Laboratory Evaluations for Integrative and Functional Medicine*, 2nd ed. Duluth: Metametrix Institute.

McCandless, Jaquelyn. 2009. *Children with Starving Brains*. Wilton Manors: Bramble.

Murray, Robert, et al. 2009. *Harper's Illustrated Biochemistry*, 28th ed. New York: McGraw-Hill Medical.

Pangborn, Jon. 2013. Nutritional Supplement Use for Autism Spectrum Disorder. San Diego: Autism Research Institute.

Walsh, William. 2012. *Nutrient Power*. New York: Skyhorse.

Diet
Elder, J. H. 2008. The Gluten-free, Casein-free Diet in Autism: An Overview with Clinical Implications. *Nutrition in Clinical Practice* 23(6):583–8.

Jyonouchi, H., S. Sun, and N. Itokazu. 2002. Innate Immunity Associated with Inflammatory Responses and Cytokine Production against Common Dietary Proteins in Patients with Autism Spectrum Disorder. *Neuropsychobiology* 46(2):76–84.

Pelsser L. M., et al. 2011. Effects of a Restricted Elimination Diet on the Behaviour of Children with Attention-Deficit Hyperactivity Disorder (INCA study): A Randomised Controlled Trial. *The Lancet*. 377(9764):494–503.

Reichelt, K. L., and A. M. Knivsberg. 2003. Can the Pathophysiology of Autism Be Explained by the Nature of the Discovered Urine Peptides? *Nutritional Neuroscience* 6(1):19–28.

Reichelt, K. L., and A. M. Knivsberg. 2009. The Possibility and Probability of a Gut-to-Brain Connection in Autism. *Annals of Clinical Psychiatry* 21(4):205–11.

Whiteley, P., et al. 2010. The ScanBrit Randomised, Controlled, Single-Blind Study of a Gluten- and Casein-free Dietary Intervention for Children with Autism Spectrum Disorders. *Nutritional Neuroscience* 13(2):87–100.

Whiteley, P., and P. Shattock. 2002. Biochemical Aspects in Autism Spectrum Disorders: Updating the Opioid-excess Theory and Presenting New Opportunities for Biomedical Intervention. *Expert Opinion on Therapeutic Targets* 6(2):175–83.

Epigenetics
Boris, M., A. Goldblatt, J. Galanko, and J. James 2004. Association of MTHFR Gene Variants with Autism. *Journal of the American Physicians and Surgeons* 9(4)106–8.

Hallmayer, J., et al. 2011. Genetic Heritability and Shared Environmental Factors among Twin Pairs with Autism. *Archives of General Psychiatry* 68(11):1095–102.

Miyake, K., et al. 2012. Epigenetics in Autism and Other Neurodevelopmental Diseases. *Advances in Experimental Medicine and Biology* 724:91–8. Review.

GI/Digestive System

Buie, T., et al. 2010. Evaluation, Diagnosis, and Treatment of Gastrointestinal Disorders in Individuals with ASDs: A Consensus Report. *Pediatrics* 125 Suppl 1:S1–18.

Buie, T., et al. 2010. Recommendations for Evaluation and Treatment of Common Gastrointestinal Problems in Children with ASDs. *Pediatrics* 125 Suppl 1:S19–29.

de Magistris, L., et al. 2010. Alterations of the Intestinal Barrier in Patients With Autism Spectrum Disorders and in Their First-degree Relatives. *Journal of Pediatric Gastroenterology and Nutrition* 51(4):418–24.

D'Eufemia, P., et al. 1996. Abnormal Intestinal Permeability in Children with Autism. *Acta Paediatrica* 85(9):1076–9.

Dysbiosis

Ackerman, J. 2012. How Bacteria in Our Bodies Protect Our Health. *Scientific American*, May 15.

Adams, J. B., et al. 2011. Gastrointestinal Flora and Gastrointestinal Status in Children with Autism—Comparisons to Typical Children and Correlation with Autism Severity. *BMC Gastroenterology* 11:22.

Critchfield, J. W., et al. 2011. The Potential Role of Probiotics in the Management of Childhood Autism Spectrum Disorders. *Gastroenterology Research and Practice* 2011:161358.

Parracho, H. M., et al. 2005. Differences between the Gut Microflora of Children with Autistic Spectrum Disorders and That of Healthy Children. *Journal of Medical Microbiology* 54(Pt 10):987–91.

Shaw, W. 2010. Increased Urinary Excretion of a 3-(3-hydroxyphenyl)-3-hydroxypropionic Acid (HPHPA), an Abnormal Phenylalanine Metabolite of Clostridia spp. in the Gastrointestinal Tract, in Urine Samples from Patients with Autism and Schizophrenia. *Nutritional Neuroscience* 13(3):135–43.

Immune System

Ashwood, P., et al. 2011. Elevated Plasma Cytokines in Autism Spectrum Disorders Provide Evidence of Immune Dysfunction and Are Associated with Impaired Behavioral Outcome. *Brain, Behavior, and Immunity* 25(1):40–5.

Cabanlit, M., et al. 2007. Brain-specific Autoantibodies in the Plasma of Subjects with Autistic Spectrum Disorder. *Annals of the New York Academy of Sciences* 1107:92–103.

Careaga, M., J. Van de Water, and P. Ashwood. 2010. Immune Dysfunction in Autism: A Pathway to Treatment. *Neurotherapeutics* 7(3):283–92.

Goines, P., et al. 2011. Autoantibodies to Cerebellum in Children with Autism Associate with Behavior. *Brain, Behavior, and Immunity* 25(3):514–23.

Heuer, L., et al. 2008. Reduced Levels of Immunoglobulin in Children with Autism Correlates with Behavioral Symptoms. *Autism Research* 1(5):275.

Zimmerman, A. W., et al. 2005. Cerebrospinal Fluid and Serum Markers of Inflammation in Autism. *Pediatric Neurology* 33(3):195.

Methylation

Deth, R., et al. 2008. How Environmental and Genetic Factors Combine to Cause Autism: A Redox/Methylation Hypothesis. *Neurotoxicology* 29(1):190–201.

James, S. J., et al. 2004. Metabolic Biomarkers of Increased Oxidative Stress and Impaired Methylation Capacity in Children with Autism. *American Journal of Clinical Nutrition* 80(6):1611–7.

Mitochondria/Energy Metabolism

Frye, R. E., and D. A. Rossignol. 2011. Mitochondrial Dysfunction Can Connect the Diverse Medical Symptoms Associated with Autism Spectrum Disorders. *Pediatric Research* 69(5 Pt 2):41R–7R.

Giulivi, C., et al. 2010. Mitochondrial Dysfunction in Autism. *Journal of the American Medical Association* 304(21):2389–96.

Melnyk, S., et al. 2012. Metabolic Imbalance Associated with Methylation Dysregulation and Oxidative Damage in Children with Autism. *Journal of Autism and Developmental Disorders* 42(3):367–77.

Rossignol, D. A., and J. J. Bradstreet. 2008. Evidence of Mitochondrial Dysfunction in Autism and Implications for Treatment. *American Journal of Biochemistry and Biotechnology* 4(2):208–17.

Rossignol, D. A., and R. E. Frye. 2012. Mitochondrial Dysfunction in Autism Spectrum Disorders: A Systematic Review and Meta-analysis. *Molecular Psychiatry* 17:290–314. doi:10.1038/mp.2010.136.

Neurology

Frye, R. E., et al. 2012 Cerebral Folate Receptor Autoantibodies in Autism Spectrum Disorder. *Molecular Psychiatry*, January 10. doi:10.1038/mp.2011.175.

Herbert, M. 2006. Autism: A Brain Disorder, or Disorder that Affects the Brain? *Clinical Neuropsychiatry* 2:354–79.

MacFabe, D. F., et al. 2007. Neurobiological Effects of Intraventricular Propionic Acid in Rats: Possible Role of Short Chain Fatty Acids on the Pathogenesis and Characteristics of Autism Spectrum Disorders. *Behavioural Brain Research* 176(1):149–69.

Mehler, M. F., and D. P. Purpura. 2009. Autism, Fever, Epigenetics and the Locus Coeruleus. *Brain Research Reviews* 59(2):388–92.

Pardo, C. A., et al. 2005. Immunity, Neuroglia and Neuroinflammation in Autism. *International Review of Psychiatry* 17(6):485–95.

Qin, L., et al. 2007. Systemic LPS Causes Chronic Neuroinflammation and Progressive Neurodegeneration. *Glia* 55(5):453–62.

Shultz, S. R., et al. 2008. Intracerebroventricular Injection of Propionic Acid, an Enteric Bacterial Metabolic End-product, Impairs Social Behavior in the Rat: Implications for an Animal Model of Autism. *Neuropharmacology* 54(6):901–11.

Singer, H. S., et al. 2006. Antibrain Antibodies in Children with Autism and Their Unaffected Siblings. *Journal of Neuroimmunology* 178(1–2):149.

Vargas, D. L., et al. 2005. Neuroglial Activation and Neuroinflammation in the Brain of Patients with Autism. *Annals of Neurology* 57(1):67–81.

Zimmerman, A. W., et al. 2007. Maternal Antibrain Antibodies in Autism. *Brain, Behavior, and Immunity* 21(3):351–7.

Nutrients and Nutritional Deficiencies

Adams, et al. 2001. Effect of a Vitamin/Mineral Supplement on Children and Adults with Autism. *BMC Pediatrics* 11:111.

Adams, et al. 2011. Nutritional and Metabolic Status of Children with Autism vs. Neurotypical Children, and the Association with Autism Severity. *Nutrition & Metabolism* 8(1):34.

Amminger, G. P., et al. 2007. Omega-3 Fatty Acids Supplementation in Children with Autism: A Double-blind Randomized, Placebo-controlled Pilot Study. *Biological Psychiatry* 61(4):551–3.

Bradstreet, J. J., et al. 2010. Biomarker-guided Interventions of Clinically Relevant Conditions Associated with Autism Spectrum Disorders and Attention Deficit Hyperactivity Disorder. *Alternative Medicine Review* 15(1):15–32.

Bilici, M., et al. 2004. Double-blind, Placebo-controlled Study of Zinc Sulfate in the Treatment of Attention Deficit Hyperactivity Disorder. *Progress in Neuropsychopharmacology and Biological Psychiatry* 28:181–90.

Curtis, L. T., and K. Patel. 2008. Nutritional and Environmental Approaches to Preventing and Treating Autism and Attention Deficit Hyperactivity Disorder (ADHD): A Review. *Journal of Alternative and Complementary Medicine* 14(1):79–85.

Jory, J., and W. R. McGinnis. 2008. Red-cell Trace Minerals in Children with Autism. *American Journal of Biochemistry and Biotechnology* 4(2):101–104.

Kałużna-Czaplińska, J. 2011. Noninvasive Urinary Organic Acids Test to Assess Biochemical and Nutritional Individuality in Autistic Children. *Clinical Biochemistry* 44(8–9):686–91.

Khan, Y., and G. Tisman. 2010. Pica in Iron Deficiency: A Case Series. *Journal of Medical Case Reports* 4:86.

Lakhan, S. E., and K. F. Vieira. 2010. Nutritional and Herbal Supplements for Anxiety and Anxiety-related Disorders: Systematic Review. *Nutrition Journal* 9:42.

Mainardi, T., S. Kapoor, and L. Bielory. 2009. Complementary and Alternative Medicine: Herbs, Phytochemicals and Vitamins and Their Immunologic Effects. *Journal of Allergy and Clinical Immunology* 123(2):283–94, quiz 295–6.

Martí, L. F. 2010. Effectiveness of Nutritional Interventions on the Functioning of Children with ADHD and/or ASD: An Updated Review of Research Evidence. *Boletín de la Asociación Médica de Puerto Rico* 102(4):31–42.

Meiri, G., et al. 2009. Omega 3 Fatty Acid Treatment in Autism. *Journal of Child and Adolescent Psychopharmacology* 19(4):449–51.

Milte, C. M., et al. 2012. Eicosapentaenoic and Docosahexaenoic Acids, Cognition, and Behavior in Children with Attention-Deficit/Hyperactivity Disorder: A Randomized Controlled Trial. *Nutrition* 28(6):670–7.

Mousain-Bosc, M., et al. 2006. Improvement of Neurobehavioral Disorders in Children Supplemented with Magnesium-Vitamin B6. II. Pervasive Developmental Disorder-Autism. *Magnesium Research* 19(1):53–62.

Richardson, A. J. 2006. Omega-3 Fatty Acids in ADHD and Related Neurodevelopmental Disorders. *International Review of Psychiatry* 18(2):155–72.

Rossignol, D. A. 2009. Novel and Emerging Treatments for Autism Spectrum Disorders: A Systematic Review. *Annals of Clinical Psychiatry* 21(4):213–36.

Sarris, J., et al. 2011. Complementary Medicines (Herbal and Nutritional Products) in the Treatment of Attention Deficit Hyperactivity Disorder (ADHD): A Systematic Review of the Evidence. *Complementary Therapies in Medicine* 19(4):216–27.

Websites

Office of Dietary Supplements, NIH. Dietary Supplement Fact Sheets: http://ods.od.nih.gov/factsheets/list-all/

University of Maryland Medical Alternative Medicine Index: www.umm.edu/altmed/

Oxidative Stress

James, S. J., et al. 2005. Thimerosal Neurotoxicity Is Associated with Glutathione Depletion: Protection with Glutathione Precursors. *Neurotoxicology* 26(1):1–8.

James, S. J., et al. 2006. Metabolic Endophenotype and Related Genotypes Are Associated with Oxidative Stress in Children with Autism. *American Journal of Medical Genetics, Part B, Neuropsychiatric Genetics* 141B(8):947–56.

James, S. J., et al. 2009. Efficacy of Methylcobalamin and Folinic Acid Treatment on Glutathione Redox Status in Children with Autism. *American Journal of Clinical Nutrition* 89(1):425–30.

Ming, X., et al. 2008. Evidence of Oxidative Stress in Autism Derived from Animal Models. *American Journal of Biochemistry and Biotechnology* 4(2):218–225.

Sulfation

Grandjean, P., and P. J. Landrigan. 2006. Developmental Neurotoxicity of Industrial Chemicals. *The Lancet.* 368(9553):2167–78.

Russo, J. P., et al. 2006. Autism and Environmental Genomics. *Neurotoxicology* 27(5):671–84.

Waring, R. H., and L. V. Klovrza. 2000. Sulphur Metabolism in Autism. *Journal of Nutritional and Environmental Medicine.* 10:25–32.

Toxins and Toxic Exposures

Adams, J. B., et al. 2009. The Severity of Autism Is Associated with Toxic Metal Body Burden and Red Blood Cell Glutathione Levels. *Journal of Toxicology* 2009:532640.

Bouchard, M. F., et al. 2010. Attention-Deficit/Hyperactivity Disorder and Urinary Metabolites of Organophosphate Pesticides. *Pediatrics* 125(6):e1270–7.

Lord, R. S., and J. A. Bralley. 2008. *Laboratory Evaluations for Integrative and Functional Medicine*, 2nd ed., 121. Duluth, GA: Metametrix Institute.

Woods, J. S., et al. 2010. Urinary Porphyrin Excretion in Neurotypical and Autistic Children. *Environmental Health Perspectives* 118(10):1450–7.

Miscellaneous

Rossignol, D. A., and R. E. Frye. 2012. A Review of Research Trends in Physiological Abnormalities in Autism Spectrum Disorders: Immune Dysregulation, Inflammation, Oxidative Stress, Mitochondrial Dysfunction and Environmental Toxicant Exposures. *Molecular Psychiatry* 17(4):389–401.

Shoffner, J., et al. 2009. Fever Plus Mitochondrial Disease Could Be Risk Factors for Autistic Regression. *Journal of Child Neurology*, September 22.

About the Authors

Dana Godbout Laake, M.S., L.D.N., is a licensed nutritionist providing preventive and therapeutic medical nutrition services through Dana Laake Nutrition in Kensington, Maryland. Her practice encompasses the full spectrum of complex health issues in all ages, including children with special needs, ADHD, and autism. An honors graduate from Temple University, she received four gubernatorial appointments to two Maryland health care regulatory and licensing boards, and served as a state legislative assistant on nutrition issues. She provides professional continuing education courses, and hosts a radio show, "Essentials of Healthy Living."

Pamela J. Compart, M.D., is a developmental pediatrician in Columbia, Maryland. She did her pediatric training at Children's National Medical Center in Washington, D.C., and fellowship training in behavioral and developmental pediatrics at the University of Maryland School of Medicine. She combines traditional and complementary medicine approaches to the treatment of ADHD, autism, and other behavioral and developmental disorders. Dietary changes and use of nutritional supplements complement traditional treatments such as appropriate educational placement and speech therapy, occupational therapy, and other therapies. She is also the founder and director of HeartLight Healing Arts, a multidisciplinary integrated holistic health care practice, providing services for children, adults, and families.

Acknowledgments

Dana Godbout Laake, R.D.H., M.S., L.D.N.

Long ago I chose the path less traveled—a fascinating journey with a fluctuating itinerary and far more sunny days than bumps along the way. It has always been the exceptional traveling companions and support team who made the adventure not only possible, but extraordinary. With deep gratitude, I thank the courageous pioneers and visionaries who prevailed against all odds, my colleagues who generously shared their knowledge, and family and friends who encourage and cheer.

- My co-author, Pam Compart, for her exceptional proficiency, insightful challenges, incredible diligence, and, most importantly, her integrity and friendship.
- William (Billy) Crook, M.D.—pediatrician whose books on yeast changed lives.
- Bernard Rimland, Ph.D.—founder of the Autism Research Institute, who shed the light on autism as a neurodevelopmental, biochemical and treatable disorder.
- Jon Pangborn, Ph.D.—author, and educator whose courses in nutritional biochemistry laid the foundation for biomedical treatments.
- Sidney McDonald Baker, M.D.—author and visionary who transformed the treatment of autism by asking, "Have we done everything we can for this child?"
- Jeffrey Bland, Ph.D.—the "Socrates of nutrition" and internationally-recognized expert in nutritional biochemistry and functional medicine.
- George Mitchell, M.D.—the mentor who introduced me to alternative medicine.
- The Autism Research Institute's Steve Edelson, Jane Johnson, Denise Fulton, and the dedicated staff and extraordinary team of brilliant professionals who make a profoundly positive difference in the lives of the community we serve: Elizabeth Mumper, Martha Herbert, Nancy O'Hara, Jill James, Dan Rossignol, Jim Adams, Richard Frye, David Berger, Judy Van de Water, Robert Naviaux, Stuart Freedenfeld, Doreen Granpeesheh, Anju Usman, and so many more.
- The best team of nutritionists and advisors: Kelly Dorfman, Victoria Wood, Kelly Barnhill, Julie Matthews, Peta Cohen, Vicki Kobliner, Liz Lipski, and Tom Malterre.
- Friends who consistently stay the course: Pam Foster, Teresa Griswold, Mary Kay Almy, Glenda Ingham, Bev Bailey, Bonnie Gutman, Pam Wilson, Pat Godbout, Jeannie Godbout, Joan Sweeney, Ann Walsh, Judy Eisenacher, and the Schmidts, Myses, and DeLawters.
- Our ever-expanding, "patchwork quilt of a family"—the Beers, Clarks, Laakes, Reddings, Browns, Wilsons, Trainers, Goffs, Kohns, and our Godbout family—from the in-laws to wonderful nieces and nephews.
- Two very special Godbouts: Christina and Michael.
- My incredibly gifted and witty sister Susan Clark, our forever brother-in-law Bill Clark, Jr., and awesome nephew, Tim Clark.
- The "son shines" of our lives, who continue to amaze and entertain us, Rich and Greg Godbout, and Pete, Jr. and Steve Laake. We are honored to be your parents.
- To our daughters-in-law, whose places in this family had long been reserved: Julie Kohn Godbout, Colleen Redding Godbout, Carron Trainer Laake, and Marisa Goff Laake.

- To our "truly grand" grandchildren who fill spaces in our hearts we never knew were empty: Peter, Kit, and Sammi Laake; Ella Godbout: Skylar Laake; and Brody Godbout.
- And always with love and gratitude to Peter Winston Laake, Sr.—my "solutions" advisor, my foundation, my husband—whose love, generosity, and wit have made all the difference. May I have this dance for the rest of my life?

Pamela J. Compart, M.D.

- To my brilliant coauthor, Dana Laake, whom I often describe to my patients as "the smartest person I know." Her intellect is only surpassed by her compassion, dedication, and generosity of spirit, and I am privileged to know and work with her.
- To my dear friend and HeartLight's nurse/nutritionist, Jennifer Sima, for her helpful contributions to the nutrient sections of this book and for her invaluable and ongoing support and friendship.
- To Dr. Elizabeth Mumper, founder and director of Advocates for Children and the Rimland Center, for her exquisite writing and contribution to this book, her dedication to her patients and the autism community, and her continual availability as a supportive colleague and adviser.
- To Dr. Carol Greene, genetic/metabolic specialist at the University of Maryland Medical Center, for always being available to answer "just one more question" about mitochondrial/metabolic issues in my patients.
- To Dr. Sidney Baker, for writing the book (*Detoxification and Healing*) that changed my entire approach to medicine, and in so doing, my career path, and for being an inspiration to all of us in this field of functional medicine.
- To the Autism Research Institute and all its speakers, researchers, and staff for their tireless dedication to continually asking new questions and seeking out new answers with both enthusiasm and scientific rigor.
- To the practitioners and staff of my practice, HeartLight Healing Arts, for inspiring me with their clinical expertise and the openness of their hearts; it is a joy to go to work every day with such dedicated and caring professionals.
- To my late parents, Ruth and Henry Compart, for always believing in me, through the various ebbs and flows of my career and life paths; there is no substitute for the love and support of parents, and I was extraordinarily blessed.
- To my brothers and sisters-in-law, for reminding me of the joys of life outside the office and for gifting me with two remarkable nephews (in my completely unbiased opinion).
- And finally, to the families, parents, and children whom I am privileged to serve: To the parents who never expected to have to be biochemists when they signed on to be parents, who do the hard work and never give up, who love their children unconditionally, and who inspire me every day. And to the children who work the hardest of all and who have such exquisite gifts that are too often hidden behind their outward symptoms. I continue to learn so much more from them than they do from me.

Index